first place 4 health

Bible Study Series

seek God first

Published by Gospel Light
Ventura, California, U.S.A.
www.gospellight.com
Printed in the U.S.A.

Library of Congress Cataloging-in-Publication Data
First Place 4 Health Bible study series : Seek God first.
p. cm.
ISBN 978-0-8307-5572-1 (trade paper)
1. Spiritual life—Christianity—Textbooks. 2. Spirituality—Textbooks.
3. Weight loss—Religious aspects—Christianity—Textbooks.
I. Gospel Light Publications (Firm)
BV4501.3.F5693 2009
248.4—dc22
2009036917

Rights for publishing this book outside the U.S.A. or in non-English
languages are administered by Gospel Light Worldwide, an international
not-for-profit ministry. For additional information, please visit
www.glww.org, email info@glww.org, or write to Gospel Light Worldwide,
1957 Eastman Avenue, Ventura, CA 93003, U.S.A.

contents

BIBLE STUDIES

ADDITIONAL MATERIALS

foreword

My introduction to Bible study came when I joined First Place in March 1981. I had been attending church since I was a small child, but the extent of my study of the Bible had been reading my Sunday School quarterly on Saturday night. On Sunday morning, I would listen to my Sunday School teacher as she taught God's Word to me. During the worship service, I would listen to our pastor as he taught God's Word to me. Frankly, the idea of digging out the truths of the Bible for myself had never entered my mind.

Perhaps you are right where I was back in 1981. If so, you are in for a blessing you never dreamed possible. As you start studying the truths of the Bible for yourself through the First Place 4 Health Bible studies, you will see God begin to open your understanding of His Word.

Almost every First Place 4 Health member I have talked with about the program says, "The weight loss is wonderful, but the most important thing I have received from my association with First Place 4 Health is learning to study God's Word." The First Place 4 Health Bible studies are designed to be done on a daily basis. As you work through each day's study (which will take 15 to 20 minutes to complete), you will be discovering the deep truths of God's Word. A part of each week's study will also include a Bible memory verse for the week.

There are many in-depth Bible studies on the market. The First Place 4 Health Bible studies are not designed for the purpose of in-depth study, but are designed to be used in conjunction with the rest of the program to bring balance into your life. Our desire is for each member to begin having a personal quiet time with God each day. This time alone with God should include a time of prayer, Bible reading and Bible study. Having a quiet time is a daily discipline that will bring the rich rewards of balance, which is something we all need.

God bless you as you begin this exciting journey toward a balanced life. God will richly bless your efforts to give Him first place in your life. Remember Matthew 6:33: "But seek first his kingdom and his righteousness, and all these things will be given to you as well."

Carole Lewis, First Place 4 Health National Director

introduction

First Place 4 Health is a Christ-centered health program that emphasizes balance in the physical, mental, emotional and spiritual areas of life. The First Place 4 Health program is meant to be a daily process. As we learn to keep Christ first in our lives, we will find that He is the One who satisfies our hunger and our every need.

This Bible study is designed to be used in conjunction with the First Place 4 Health program but can be beneficial for anyone interested in obtaining a balanced lifestyle. The Bible study has been created in a five-day format, with the last two days reserved for reflection on the material studied. Keep in mind that the ultimate goal of studying the Bible is not only for knowledge but also for application and a changed life. Don't feel anxious if you can't seem to find the *correct* answer. Many times, the Word will speak differently to different people, depending on where they are in their walk with God and the season of life they are experiencing. Be prepared to discuss with your fellow First Place 4 Health members what you learned that week through your study.

There are some additional components included with this study that will be helpful as you pursue the goal of giving Christ first place in every area of your life:

- **Group Prayer Request Form:** This form is at the end of each week's study. You can use this to record any special requests that might be given in class.

- **Leader Discussion Guide:** This discussion guide is provided to help the First Place 4 Health leader guide a group through this Bible study. It includes ideas for facilitating a First Place 4 Health class discussion for each week of the Bible study.

- **Two Weeks of Menu Plans with Recipes:** There are 14 days of meals, and all are interchangeable. Each day totals 1,400 to 1,500 calories and includes snacks. Instructions are given for those who need more calories. An accompanying grocery list includes items needed for each week of meals.

- **First Place 4 Health Member Survey:** Fill this out and bring it to your first meeting. This information will help your leader know your interests and talents.

- **Personal Weight and Measurement Record:** Use this form to keep a record of your weight loss. Record any loss or gain on the chart after the weigh-in at each week's meeting.

- **Weekly Prayer Partner Forms:** Fill out this form before class and place it into a basket during the class meeting. After class, you will draw out a prayer request form, and this will be your prayer partner for the week. Try to call or email the person sometime before the next class meeting to encourage that person.

- **Live It Trackers:** Your Live It Tracker is to be completed at home and turned in to your leader at your weekly First Place 4 Health meeting. The Tracker is designed to help you practice mindfulness and stay accountable with regard to your eating and exercise habits. Step-by-step instructions for how to use the Live It Tracker are provided in the *Member's Guide*.

- **Let's Count Our Miles!** A worthy goal we encourage is for you to complete 100 miles of exercise during your 12 weeks in First Place 4 Health. There are many activities listed on pages 255-256 that count toward your goal of 100 miles. When you complete a mile of activity, mark off the box listed on the Hundred Mile Club chart located on the inside of the back cover.

- **Scripture Memory Cards:** These cards have been designed so you can use them while exercising. It is suggested that you punch a hole in the upper left corner and place the cards on a ring. You may want to take the cards in the car or to work so you can practice each week's Scripture memory verse throughout the day.

- **Scripture Memory CD:** All 10 Scripture memory verses have been put to music at an exercise tempo in the CD at the back of this study. Use this CD when exercising or even when you are just driving in your car. The words of Scripture are often easier to memorize when accompanied by music.

welcome to
Seek God First

At your first group meeting for this session of First Place 4 Health, you will meet your fellow members, get an overview of your materials and find out what you can expect at weekly meetings. The majority of your class time will be spent learning about the four-sided person concept, the Live It Food Plan, and how change begins from the inside out. You will also have a chance to ask any questions about how to get the most out of First Place 4 Health. If possible, complete the Member Survey on page 205 before your first group meeting. The information that you give will help your leader tailor the next 12 weeks to the needs of the whole group.

Each weekly meeting begins with a weigh-in for members. This will allow you to track your progress over the 12-week session. Your Week One weigh-in/measurement will establish a baseline of comparison so that you can set healthy goals for this session. If you are apprehensive about weighing in every week, talk with your group leader about your concerns. He or she will have some options for you to consider that will make the weigh-in activity encouraging rather than stressful.

The day after your first meeting, begin Week Two of this Bible study. This session, you and your group will explore the importance of centering your goals for a healthy life on Jesus. No matter how strong your body, mind and emotions may appear, unless you have spiritual tenacity and re-solve, you will not be able to run the course God has laid out for you. As you open yourself to the truth of Scripture and share your hopes and struggles with the members of your group during the next 12 weeks, you'll find yourself becoming the healthy child of God you are designed to be!

Week Two

first things first

SCRIPTURE MEMORY VERSE
*But seek first his kingdom and his righteousness,
and all these things will be given to you as well.*
MATTHEW 6:33

When asked by the religious leaders of His day what was the greatest commandment, Jesus answered, "Love the Lord your God with all your heart and with all your soul and with all your mind and with all your strength" (Mark 12:30). Our Creator fashioned us as multi-faceted beings: people with a wonderfully made body, an intricate mind, a wide range of emotions—and a spiritual dimension as well. All of these aspects of our being (emotional, spiritual, intellectual and physical) need to be brought into balance in order for us to attain our full potential as humans created to glorify God. Only when we are leading a balanced life in all four areas will we be restored to the health and wholeness that honors our Creator.

Matthew 6:33 gives us a pattern for living this kind of Christ-centered life: We learn to seek His kingdom and His righteousness *first* in our lives. We begin each day with a multitude of choices to make. Some choices are the mundane daily ones: what to wear, what to eat, when to do the laundry or vacuum the house, whether to take the bus or walk to work. Other choices may be more important: whether or not to confront your spouse (or child or boss) about a problem, deciding whether to choose surgery over alternative medical procedures, choosing a church that you and your family can call home. As you begin each day, choosing to seek His kingdom and His righteousness first will center the other choices you make on God's will and will put you on the right track in all the other areas of your life.

This week's study will lead you in making Christ-honoring choices that will have an eternal impact on all four aspects of your life.

SEEK CHRIST FIRST

Day
1

Almighty God, help me to choose Your path for my life today. Empower me through Your Holy Spirit to make the commitments to live a healthy balanced life, centered on Jesus Christ, my Lord and Savior. Amen.

This week's memory verse is found in the midst of Jesus' Sermon on the Mount (see Matthew 5–7), a discourse in which Jesus outlined several principles for the people of His day to live radically different lives. Imagine for a moment the people who were listening to the words He so profoundly spoke. They were struggling to survive in a land occupied by Rome, a fearfully powerful government, and had little or no control of their own lives. And yet, in the midst of this sermon, Jesus instructed them to seek God's kingdom and righteousness and all their needs would be met! Their physical needs were simple: food, water, shelter and clothing. We have those same needs today, but in our culture few of us actually are in desperate need of these basics. However, there are emotional, spiritual, physical and intellectual needs that impact our lives.

As you begin today's study, take a quick look at the entries in your calendar or your checkbook for the past month. What areas have you been giving first place in your life? To which areas are you devoting the most time and effort?

Read Matthew 6:25-30. What are some of the concerns that divert our attention from Jesus' priorities in our lives (see v. 25)?

_____

_____

_____

Across this list, write in large letters what Jesus instructs us *not* to do about these concerns. What does this verse tell you about God's understanding of your needs?

_____

_____

_____

_____

Jesus wasn't saying that these things are not important, but He does instruct us not to worry about them. These concerns do not need to be the focus of our daily existence. What does Matthew 6:26-30 teach us about God's loving care for us?

_____

_____

_____

What promise is found in Philippians 4:19? Do you believe this promise applies to you?

_____

_____

_____

As you embark on this journey to a healthier lifestyle, consider the goals you might have for the four aspects of your life. Place a check beside the aspect(s) that most concerns you. Pray about your concerns, and then write one specific step you could make to begin to achieve this goal in your life. For example, perhaps you are concerned about adding more time for exercise in your already jam-packed schedule. You could begin to add more exercise to your routine by planning to park a little farther from your workplace or shopping destination. Make your goals reasonable and attainable.

☐ Emotional (heart)

_____

_____

_____

☐ Spiritual (soul)

_____

_____

_____

☐ Mental (mind)

_____

_____

_____

☐ Physical (body)

_____

_____

_____

As Christians, the desire to give Christ first place in every area of our lives must be foremost. *Saying* Christ is first and *living* with Christ in first place are two different matters. When Christ enters our lives, our lives will change. We will make new decisions based on new commitments. We will schedule our time based on new priorities.

Thank You, Lord, for Your promise to meet my needs. Help me to trust You for those needs and to give You first place in my life today. Amen.

PUT ASIDE WORRY

Heavenly Father, thank You that I can trust You to provide what I need. Help me, Lord, to put my focus on You and Your provision for this day. Amen.

As we learned in yesterday's study, God has promised that we will receive what we need. In spite of this, most Christians continue to worry rather than simply claim this promise. Worry is an affront to God—we might even say a sin! He told us He would supply all our needs, and He knows what we need even before we ask.

In Matthew 6:28-34, Jesus continues to teach about not worrying over the needs of life. Worry is different from being concerned. God wants you to be concerned to the point of placing circumstances in His hands, seeing a need and taking care of the needs of others. Pray earnestly about those things, but don't worry and fret over them. Many times, the things that we worry about either never happen or they are things over which we have no control.

What are the things that cause you worry? How much time and energy do you spend worrying about these things each week? What is the percentage of this list of worries over which you have no control?

_____

_____

_____

_____

Putting aside worry may seem to be easier said than done, but one of the best ways to rid yourself of a bad habit is to replace that habit with a positive action. According to Philippians 4:6, what is a positive action that you can take when you find yourself worrying about something?

_____

_____

_____

_____

What is the positive outcome found in verse 7?

_____

_____

_____

How would your life change if you invested your emotional energy in spiritual priorities rather than on worrying?

_____

_____

_____

It may seem simplistic to say that we can pray and our worries will dissolve, but in John 14:14 we find a wonderful promise from Jesus. Write that promise here.

_____

_____

_____

When you pray about the things that cause you to worry and you believe in God's faithfulness, He will provide what you need—whether that need is the basics of food and shelter or the need to trust your heavenly Father to take away the temptation to worry. Make a list of the circumstances or situations in your life right now that are causing you to worry.

_____

_____

_____

_____

As you complete today's study, list in your prayer journal the details of your worries. Now write a prayer, turning each of your worries over to Him. Repeat this week's memory verse in your prayer, telling God you are willing to seek His kingdom first and trust Him to provide whatever you need.

Lord, help me to seek You and Your kingdom first and to put my trust in You. Remind me to focus my energy on things that will make a difference for Your kingdom. Thank You for Your peace that surpasses all understanding. Amen.

Day 3 — SET THE RIGHT PRIORITIES

Heavenly Father, thank You that You have made me a part of Your kingdom. Help me to better understand what that means in my life. Amen.

When Jesus told His listeners to seek God's kingdom and "all these things will be given to you as well" (Matthew 6:33), He was referring to what He had previously discussed: "your life, what you will eat or drink . . . your body, what you will wear" (v. 25). In other words, He was speaking of the basic necessities of life. In making this statement, Jesus was basically saying that we can choose to worry about these things or we can seek God's kingdom and rest in the knowledge that God will take care of us. The choice is ours.

Read Matthew 6:9-13. What does verse 10 say about God's kingdom?

_____

_____

_____

In Romans 14:17, what two things are listed that *are not* priorities in the kingdom of God?

1. _____

2. _____

What three things *are* priorities in the kingdom of God?

1. _____

2. _____

3. _____

Notice that the two items listed in Romans 14:17 that are not priorities in the kingdom of God concern our *physical* lives, while the three items listed that are priorities concern our *spiritual* lives. Of course, this does not mean that our physical needs are unimportant. What do the following verses tell us about taking care of responsibilities and physical needs?

2 Thessalonians 3:10

_____

_____

_____

1 Timothy 5:8

_____

_____

_____

While spiritual priorities must be foremost, we also need to provide for our own physical needs and those of others. The challenge is to live responsibly without allowing daily pressures to consume most of our time and energy. What does Psalm 37:4 tell us about focusing on the Lord? What is the promise if we do this?

_____

_____

_____

In 1 Corinthians 10:31 and Colossians 3:23-24, Paul provides some guidance for transforming everyday responsibilities into a life focused on God and spiritual priorities. What should be your focus as you pursue your daily activities? What does "for the glory of God" mean to you?

_____

_____

_____

How can your participation in First Place 4 Health bring glory to God?

_____

_____

_____

Lord, without You at the center of my life, I can accomplish nothing of eternal value. Strengthen me today so I might do Your will and glorify You. Amen.

Day 4 — FOCUS ON HIS RIGHTEOUSNESS

Lord, without Your sacrifice for my sin, I could never be considered righteous. Help me to understand Your gift of righteousness as I study Your Word today.

In Titus 3:3, Paul tells us that before we came to Christ, we were "enslaved by all kinds of passions and pleasures." But then Jesus saved us and brought us into a new life. The old life passed away, and as we began to seek first the kingdom of God and His righteousness, we embraced the new priorities that Jesus had given us. Today, He lives within us and continues to play a vital role in our efforts to live a life pleasing to God.

In ancient Israel, the high priest alone could offer sacrifices to God to atone for the sins of the priests, the people and himself. Read Hebrews 5:1-3. What qualities did the high priests have? Why were they able to deal gently with those who went astray?

_____

_____

_____

Turn to Hebrews 4:14-16. How does the fact that Jesus fulfills this role of our high priest benefit us?

_____

_____

_____

What makes Jesus Christ different from the priests who ministered to God's people in the past? Why is this important? What does this enable our high priest to do for us?

In Hebrews 4:15, we read that Jesus was tempted in every way, just as we are. Because of this, He understands our weaknesses and will never chide or scold us when we come to Him. What can we thus expect from Him in our time of need?

Read Hebrews 5:7-10. Jesus was obedient and put the will of the Father first, and because of this He was "made perfect." What did His obedience enable Him to do for us?

What does this tell you about the importance of putting Christ in first place in your life?

How can you relate what you've learned about Christ's righteousness to your First Place 4 Health goals? How can your goals honor His work of righteousness for you?

In your prayer journal, write out a prayer of thanksgiving and praise to the Lord for what He has done for you through the death and resurrection of our Savior and Lord Jesus Christ.

> *God, show me how to please You in everything I do, and strengthen me when I falter from the path You have set before me. I can do nothing without the power of Your Holy Spirit within me. Amen.*

Day 5

GIVE CHRIST FIRST PLACE

Almighty God, You alone are righteous. You are worthy of all praise, honor and glory. Help me put You in first place so that my life will become balanced and focused. Amen.

In Matthew 5:14,16, Jesus told His followers, "You are the light of the world. A city on a hill cannot be hidden. Let your light shine before men, that they may see your good deeds and praise your Father in heaven." When you put Christ first in everything you do, a natural result is that others are able to see His presence in your life. The light of Christ that is within you will naturally shine out and affect all those around you. Your life becomes balanced, and your priorities are set in the proper order.

According to the following verses, what are some other attributes of one who places the Lord first?

1 Samuel 15:22

_____

_____

_____

Romans 12:1

_____

_____

_____

Romans 13:8

_____
_____
_____
_____

2 Corinthians 9:7

_____
_____
_____
_____

1 Thessalonians 5:17

_____
_____
_____
_____

Now put an *X* on the line next to each of the following statements to indicate where you are in giving Christ first place in these areas of your life:

Characteristic in My Life	Strong	Average	Weak
I desire to know and obey God.			
I offer myself to God as a living sacrifice.			
I give to God from my material possessions.			
I continually show God's love to others.			
I sustain a lifestyle of prayer.			

How can your participation in First Place 4 Health bring glory to God?

_____
_____
_____

What can you do to be instruments of encouragement for other members in your First Place 4 Health group?

_____

_____

_____

_____

How is Philippians 4:13 an encouragement to you as you seek to put His kingdom and righteousness first in your life?

_____

_____

_____

_____

Heavenly Father, help me to live today so that others might see You in my life. Allow me to be Your shining light and remind me to give all praise and glory to You alone! Give me boldness to declare Your gospel message to others when they ask. Amen.

Day 6 — REFLECTION AND APPLICATION

Lord, I choose to seek Your kingdom and Your righteousness today. Help me today to put You first in every area of my life. Amen.

Studying the Bible may be a new experience for you, or it may already be a daily part of your life. In either case, participating in the First Place 4 Health Bible studies will help you keep your spiritual priorities as well as your physical, mental and emotional needs in balance. These studies will also guide, strengthen and encourage you as you live out your life for Christ. As the title of today's and tomorrow's sessions indicate, Days 6 and 7 of each week's study are intended to help you reflect on what you have learned and then guide you in applying it to your specific situation.

What things have you learned this week about putting Christ in first place in each of the following aspects of your life?

Physical	Mental
Spiritual	Emotional

Which area do you find is your strength? Where is there room for growth in this area of strength?

_____

_____

_____

How have you been encouraged in an area of weakness this week?

_____

_____

_____

What Scripture passage has been particularly meaningful for you?

_____

_____

_____

Have you been able to encourage another group member this week? If not, how could you encourage someone right now?

_____

_____

_____

How has someone encouraged you?

_____

_____

_____

As you complete this first week of Bible study, repeat the memory verse. Keep your Scripture memory cards close at hand to help you review. Try saying the verse aloud to a family member or use it in conversation. Each time you use the verse, God will plant this verse more firmly in your mind and heart.

> *Lord, help me remember the lessons I have learned this week.*
> *Keep my heart and mind teachable and sensitive to the leading of Your*
> *Holy Spirit. Thank You for Your Word. Amen.*

Day
7

REFLECTION AND APPLICATION

Father God, You have promised to provide everything I need as I put Your kingdom and Your righteousness in first place. Strengthen my faith in Your promises and help me to live in a way that glorifies You. Amen.

One thing that will keep us from moving forward in our spiritual growth is a stronghold. In Beth Moore's book *Praying God's Word*, she explains that a stronghold may be an addiction, an unforgiving spirit toward a person who has hurt us, grief over a loss—anything that demands too much of our emotional and mental energy so that our abundant life is strangled.[1] God's Word has the power to break down those spiritual strongholds in our lives, and learning to pray through the Scriptures is a tool that can help us in that process.

Second Corinthians 10:3-5 describes our struggle and the weapons we have at our disposal to fight this battle. Reflect on these verses for a few minutes and then carefully consider the meanings of these words. You can pray this Scripture by saying something like this:

Lord, You've said I live in the world, but I do not wage war as the world does. My weapons are not the weapons of the world but have divine power to demolish strongholds. I demolish arguments and every pretension that sets itself up against the knowledge of God, and I take captive every thought to make it obedient to Christ. Thank You for working in my life. Amen.

Before we can tackle the spiritual strongholds in our lives, we need to identify the battlefield. Our mind is the control center of our being and the battlefield on which we must wage war against our enemy. Satan is our enemy, and his goal is to make us believe he is powerful and we are powerless. His weapons are the destructive and discouraging thoughts in our minds. However, we are not powerless when we have God's Holy Spirit living within us. The strongest addiction or the worst habit can be overcome through the power of the living God. Nothing is more powerful than God!

The journey to seek God's kingdom and righteousness *first* begins with a single step. The completion of this week's study is a step of progress on that journey. Rejoice in your opportunity to give Christ first place.

Father God, help me to keep in mind that my struggle is not against flesh and blood but against the rulers, against the powers of this dark world, and against the spiritual forces of evil in the heavenly realms (see Ephesians 6:12).

Lord, I have nothing to fear from my strongholds because You have given me a spirit of power and of love and of a sound mind (see 2 Timothy 1:7).

Lord, help me to be sober and vigilant, because the devil walks around like a lion, seeking whom he may devour. Help me be steadfast (see 1 Peter 5:8).

Heavenly Father, I long for You to be first in my life. I want to seek first Your kingdom and Your righteousness. Thank You for Your promise to give me the other things I need (see Matthew 6:33). Amen!

Note
1. Beth Moore, *Praying God's Word* (Nashville, TN: Broadman & Holman, 2000)

Group Prayer Requests

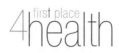

Today's Date: _____

Name	Request

Results

_____

_____

_____

_____

_____

_____

let's
pray

Last week, we examined how we need to make God's kingdom and righteousness the focus of each day. When we do so, He will provide what we need. One of the ways we can seek His will for our lives each day is through the study of His Word—the Bible. Another vital part in strengthening our spiritual life is through prayer.

Prayer is a mystery for most of us. Some people might ask, "If God knows our every need and will provide it for us, then why do we even need to *ask* Him for it?" Others struggle with how to pray, especially when they hear others pray beautiful prayers with all the *right* words, causing them to feel inadequate to come before the holy God of the universe and speak to Him of their desires, failures and need for His help. Yet our Creator has provided us with examples of prayer in His Word to help us learn to communicate with Him. And, most amazing of all, He wants us to spend time with Him in prayer.

Jesus' disciples observed that His prayers were more powerful and more effective than any prayer they had heard before. At one point, they came to Him and requested that He teach them to pray (see Luke 11:1). He responded with a model prayer—what we today call the Lord's Prayer (this prayer is recorded in Luke 11:2-4 with an expanded version recorded in Matthew 6:9-13). Notice that nowhere is it recorded that Jesus rebuked

His disciples for asking Him to teach them to pray. He simply gave them this example of prayer.

Our Creator desires to spend time in direct communication with each of us, so in His Word He has given us instructions on how to do this. In this week's study, we will learn more about who God is and how He communicates with us. We will look at models for praying, how to pray, why we pray and how prayers are answered.

Day 1 — ADORATION

Heavenly Father, make me aware of Your holiness today. Draw me close to You as I study Your Word. Teach me to pray more effectively. Amen.

We have a holy God who desires a personal relationship with us. Do you understand what an earth-shattering concept that is? No other world religion can claim that their God wants to have a personal relationship with individual believers. This week's memory verse states that "if you believe, you will receive whatever you ask for in prayer." But in what do we place our belief? In order to understand the power of prayer, we need to understand the One behind that power.

Read the model for prayer that Jesus taught His disciples in Matthew 6:9-13. What does verse 9 tell us about God?

Look up "hallowed" in a dictionary and write the definition below.

Read Isaiah 6:1-7. What comes to mind when you read this description of the holiness of the almighty God?

_____

_____

_____

According to Ephesians 2:18; 3:11-12; Hebrews 4:16 and 10:19-23, why can we approach the throne of our most holy God in prayerful confidence?

_____

_____

_____

This week's memory verse emphasizes the importance of faith/belief in the process of prayer. What does Hebrews 11:6 say about belief? What is the reward for our faith in God?

_____

_____

_____

Mark 9:17-29 tells the story of one man's encounter with Jesus that tested his faith in a healing that seemed impossible. What was the man's response to Jesus' statement "Everything is possible for him who believes" (v. 24)? What was the result of his honest statement about his faith?

_____

_____

_____

In which of your First Place 4 Health goals do you need to believe that God can accomplish the impossible? Write your need, and then follow it by writing down the man's statement from Mark 9:24.

_____

_____

_____

What does Mark 11:22-24 say about belief and doubt?

_____

_____

_____

You can pray with confidence because you have a powerful God who loves you. When you place your faith in God, your faith is based on a strong foundation.

Lord, You are faithful to keep Your promises. Help me when my faith falters and strengthen my belief in Your faithfulness to answer my prayers. Amen.

Day 2

SURRENDER

Lord, it amazes me that You want to spend time in communicating with me. Help me to learn about the process of prayer and apply it to my life. Amen.

Jesus is our example for how to live out the Christian life here on earth. The Gospels record some examples of the times and places that Jesus prayed. Read the following Scripture passages and then summarize where, when (what time of day) and what had taken place just before each time Jesus prayed. You might need to scan a few verses before or after each reference to get the context of the situation.

Verse	Where	When	Circumstances
Matt. 14:23			
Mark 1:35			
Luke 3:21			
Luke 22:41			

Summarize what you found in these verses about Jesus' habits of prayer.

_____

_____

_____

People seemed to always be demanding Jesus' time and attention, so when Jesus wanted to pray, He needed to find a place where He could be alone. Do you have a place set aside where you can meet God in prayer on a daily basis? Where is this place? If you do not presently have a place to pray in solitude, where could you do that?

_____

_____

_____

It is important to find time each day to spend in prayer. For some this might be in the early morning, for some it might be at lunchtime, and for some it might be shortly after dinner or just before bedtime. If this is not a daily habit yet for you, now is the time to make that commitment. Do you have a specific time each day for a concentrated time in communicating with the Lord in prayer? If so, when is that time?

_____

_____

_____

In Mark 1:21-34, we read what happened during the day up to verse 35. Read the passage and then write down the events that occurred:

Verses	Event(s) that Occurred
1:21 22	
1:23-26	

Verses	Event(s) that Occurred
1:29-31	
1:32-34	

Immediately after performing these miracles, Jesus went to a solitary place to pray. What does this tell you about the importance of prayer?

_____

_____

_____

Three of the four Gospels record examples of Jesus praying. Let's look at one example in Matthew 26:36-45 when Jesus was praying in the Garden of Gethsemane just before His crucifixion. How many times did Jesus pray? For what did He pray?

_____

_____

_____

Jesus was aware of the pain and humiliation that He was about to endure. He knew His heavenly Father had the power to stop the events that were set in motion. He also knew that what He was about to face had the goal to bring salvation to humankind. Jesus prayed, "Yet not as I will, but as you will," and put His life in the Father's hands. What is the promise we have in 1 John 5:14-15?

_____

_____

_____

Precious Lord, I commit myself to daily prayer, seeking Your will in my life rather than my own. Please make me aware of the obstacles that hinder my daily prayer time and help me to overcome them. Amen.

SUPPLICATION

Heavenly Father, please give me this day my daily bread.
Help me, Lord, to learn the lesson You want to teach me today. Amen.

Although many people believe that supplication (or seeking help) is the primary purpose of prayer, it is only one of many aspects. We need to be careful when we pray that we are not just treating our heavenly Father—the almighty God and creator of the universe—as our personal supernatural Santa Claus and only spend time in prayer when we need something from Him. God loves us and wants us to ask for His provision and guidance.

God has provided guidelines for our prayers of supplication. What three actions does Jesus instruct us to take in Matthew 7:7-8?

1. _____

2. _____

3. _____

What does Matthew 7:9-11 tell us about God's desire for us to ask, seek and knock?

_____

_____

_____

_____

God loves us so much that He wants us to ask for what we need and desire. How should that affect your prayer life? Is there anything too big or too small to ask of God? How can you know for sure?

_____

_____

_____

_____

Let's explore a little more about the process of asking. What do the following verses say about asking God to meet our needs?

Matthew 21:22

_____

_____

_____

John 14:13-14

_____

_____

_____

Many interpret the instruction in John 14:14 to mean that we must end each prayer by tacking on a phrase such as "in Jesus' name we pray, amen." However, this has a deeper meaning. According to the following verses, what is the additional condition to receiving what we ask for?

John 15:7

_____

_____

_____

John 15:16

_____

_____

_____

What might it mean to ask for something in Jesus' name and to trust that our request will be granted?

_____

_____

_____

In Matthew 7:7 we are instructed to "seek." But what are we to seek? Last week's memory verse gives instruction in this. Write the verse below, and then underline what we are to seek.

_____

_____

_____

_____

Luke 11:5-13 relates another version of the "ask, seek, knock" teaching. What does the word "knock" seem to indicate in his passage as it relates to praying?

_____

_____

_____

_____

Our heavenly Father wants us to *ask* for what we need (and even desire), to *seek* His holy presence, His kingdom and His righteousness, and to *knock* persistently in prayer. It is through prayer that we will come to know and understand Him more, and then we will ask in accordance with His will.

> *Dear Lord, today, I ask You not only to meet my physical needs but also to provide me with all I will need to live this day in tune with You and serve in a way that will glorify You. Amen.*

CONFESSION

Day 4

> *Heavenly Father, forgive my debts as I have also forgiven my debtors. Help me, Lord, to understand the need for daily confession and forgiveness in my prayer life. Show me what I need to confess and who I need to forgive. Amen.*

This week, we have been looking at how the Lord's Prayer provides a model for us to use in how to pray. As we have seen, this model prayer includes examples of adoration, surrender and supplication. Today, we will study how adding the key ingredients of confession and forgiveness can aid us in praying effectively.

Without looking back at the beginning of this week's study, write out this week's memory verse.

_____

_____

_____

_____

Does God really always answer our prayers? He does. Sometimes His answer is "yes," sometimes it is "no," and other times it might be "wait." However, there are certain conditions that might block us in receiving answers to our prayers. Read the following verses and summarize what each says about how to receive answers to our prayers:

James 1:5-8

_____

_____

_____

_____

James 4:3

_____

_____

_____

_____

What prayers have you prayed that have not been answered? Is there anything that you are doing or not doing that might be blocking the answers?

_____

_____

_____

One major reason for unanswered prayer might be unconfessed sin in your life. What does James 5:16 say about effective prayer?

_____

_____

_____

Some might protest that they have not sinned, but we are constantly in a struggle with our old sinful nature. What does 1 John 1:5-8 say about this? What is the solution to the problem in verse 9?

_____

_____

_____

Our prayer time should begin with a time of confession to the Lord in order to give us a clean slate to pray more effectively. Yet there is another element to consider that might be affecting our prayers: an attitude of unforgiveness. When we are unforgiving toward someone who has hurt us, it causes bitterness to take root in our lives, which adversely affects our spiritual, physical, emotional and mental health. Match the following verses with what they say about forgiveness:

____ Matthew 18:21-22   a. Forgive others to be forgiven by God.
____ Matthew 18:23-35   b. Forgive as the Lord forgave you.
____ Mark 11:23-25   c. Keep on forgiving.
____ Ephesians 4:32   d. Forgive so that the heavenly Father will forgive you.
____ Colossains 3:13   e. Forgive one another just as we are forgiven by God through Christ.

Are you harboring an unforgiving spirit toward someone who has hurt you? Even though you might have a legitimate reason to be hurt and unforgiving, you need to bring it to the Lord each time those feelings return and ask Him to help you to forgive that person. On a separate sheet of paper, write a prayer confessing your sins and/or anyone you need to forgive.

Then write 1 John 1:9 across your confession and pray with thanksgiving for God to cleanse you from all unrighteousness. When you are done, destroy the sheet of paper as a symbol of what God does for you concerning your sin and unforgiving attitude.

> *Father, help me to see that I am building a wall between You and me when I allow an attitude of unforgiveness to fester in me. Thank You, O Lord, that You have paid the price for my sins and that I need not live in that sin anymore. Amen.*

Day 5 — PROTECTION

Almighty God, do not let me yield to temptation, but deliver me from the evil one. Amen.

Some might ask, "Why do we need to pray that God will not lead us into temptation?" After all, what does James 1:13 say about God in regard to temptation?

_____

_____

_____

_____

There appears to be a contradiction here: On the one hand, Jesus seems to be telling us that we need to pray that God will not lead us into temptation; but on the other hand, James is stating that God never tempts anyone. In this instance, examining a different translation can be helpful. Matthew 6:13 in the *New Living Translation* reads, "And don't let us yield to temptation, but rescue us from the evil one." What light does this shed on the issue? What is Jesus really saying to us here?

_____

_____

_____

What does 1 Peter 2:11 say about our sinful nature?

_____

_____

_____

_____

We need to recognize how temptation may lead to sin. What is the warning found in James 1:14-15?

_____

_____

_____

_____

We are not alone in this battle against temptation. What is the promise found in Hebrews 4:15-16?

_____

_____

_____

_____

Besides the war we wage with our own sinful natures, we have another enemy who will use temptation to draw us away from God. According to Matthew 4:1-11, who is our enemy and what tactics does he use?

_____

_____

_____

_____

In Ephesians 6:13-18, Paul states that God has provided us with protective elements to help us wage war with our enemy, the devil. What has our heavenly Father provided for us as listed in these verses?

The _____ buckled around your waist (v. 14)

The _____ in place (v. 14)

Feet fitted with the _____ that comes from _____ (v. 15)

Take up the _____ (v. 16)

Take the _____ (v. 17)

and the _____, which is the Word of God (v. 17)

And _____ on all occasions (v. 18)

How can Romans 8:35-39 provide encouragement to us as we prepare to do spiritual battle?

_____

_____

_____

God, thank You for giving us a way out of the sin that entraps us. Help me to rely on You to lead me out of temptation. Thank You for the spiritual weapons You have given me to wage war against our enemy, the devil. Amen.

Day 6 REFLECTION AND APPLICATION

Our Father who is in heaven, hallowed be Your name. Your kingdom come, Your will be done on earth as it is in heaven. Amen.

We have spent the last five days learning about prayer. Do you now see that God wants to talk with you more than you could ever want to pray? Sometimes, the words will come out easily as you pray. At other times, especially in times of difficulty, you may not know what to say or how to pray. But God has made a provision for us even in those instances.

When we can't seem to find the words to pray, God provides an intercessor for us on our behalf: "The Spirit helps us in our weakness. We do not know what we ought to pray for, but the Spirit himself intercedes for us with groans that words cannot express. And he who searches our hearts knows the mind of the Spirit because the Spirit intercedes for the saints in accordance with God's will" (Romans 8:26-27).

As we have seen this week, the Lord's Prayer provides us with a pattern for our prayers: adoration, surrender, supplication, confession and protection. Although our prayers need not specifically follow this order, we need to remember these elements as we pray.

We have a creative God, and we can be creative in our communication with Him. Our prayers would become stale and merely a duty if we just stuck to the same formula each time we prayed. One way to creatively apply the principles of prayer that we have learned these last few days is to sing a praise song or read a hymn as poetry to the Lord. Another way might be to pray as you walk. After all, how can you *not* praise the Lord when you are out and walking around in His beautiful creation?

You might even want to try using different postures when you pray, such as sitting, standing, lying on your face, kneeling, or even dancing or running. Some other ideas to try might include:

- Reading prayers from the Bible or from a devotional book
- Praying with your eyes open toward heaven
- Praying with your arms uplifted
- Praying silently
- Praying aloud
- Writing your prayers in your prayer journal
- Praying in a group with others on regular occasions

What is one idea of these that are listed—or one of your own—that you might try that you've never tried before?

_____

_____

_____

_____

"O Lord, our Lord, how majestic is Your name in all the earth" (Psalm 8:1). Help me, O God, to seek You every day and to grow in wisdom. Keep me from temptation and protect me from the arrows of our enemy, the devil. Amen.

REFLECTION AND APPLICATION

Thank You, Lord, that You promise to always be near me. You promise Your peace that passes all understanding and guards my heart and my mind in Christ Jesus (see Philippians 4:5-7). Amen.

Last week, we looked at the concept of using the words of Scripture in our prayers to the Lord. This is a helpful practice that can aid us during those times when our finite human minds do not know how to pray. God has provided His Word to guide us in learning to pray effectively, and as you add to your Scripture memory bank each week by memorizing the weekly Scripture verses, you will fill your prayer arsenal to help you live righteously. Write a prayer below using this week's memory verse.

_____

_____

_____

_____

_____

_____

One aspect of prayer that we haven't yet discussed is the power that comes from corporate prayer. James 5:16 reminds us of the importance of praying for one another: "Therefore confess your sins to each other and pray for each other so that you may be healed. The prayer of a righteous man is powerful and effective."

Praying with others in your First Place 4 Health group can help you to meet the demands of daily living, and knowing that others are praying for you will give you peace and comfort during troubled times. Praying for others also has the added benefit of taking your focus off your own troubles. Remember to pray for your group members' needs each day. God wants you to be balanced emotionally, physically, mentally and spiritually. Using His Word to pray through memorized Scripture will strengthen your prayer life and help you meet the challenges and opportunities that come to you each day.

In the Ephesians 6:10-18 passage in which Paul discusses the armor of God, he lists only one offensive weapon for us to use against the enemy: the "sword of the Spirit." What does that tell us about the importance of knowing Scripture?

_____

_____

_____

_____

_____

Using Scripture in prayer will put to use the weapons of warfare and meet the conditions of prayer. Delighting yourself in the Lord and committing your way to Him by using His Word when you pray will give you the answers you seek. God answers all prayers. So humble yourself, pray, seek His face and turn from any sin in your life. Then He will hear from heaven and heal you (see 2 Chronicles 7:14).

> *Answer me when I call to You, O my righteous God. Give me relief from my distress and be merciful to me. Hear my prayer, O Lord Most High (see Psalm 4:1).*

> *Lord God, I know that without faith it is impossible to please You. I believe in You and I know that You will reward those who earnestly seek You. Help me to seek You with all my heart and soul (see Hebrews 11:6).*

> *Heavenly Father, I claim Your promise that if I pray believing that You will provide what I need, I will receive whatever I ask for in prayer. Help me to always seek Your will when I pray (see Matthew 21:22).*

Group Prayer Requests

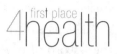

Today's Date: _____

Name	Request

Results

_____
_____
_____
_____
_____
_____

blessed
obedience

SCRIPTURE MEMORY VERSE

Whoever has my commands and obeys them, he is the one who loves me. He who loves me will be loved by my Father, and I too will love him and show myself to him.

JOHN 14:21

When you hear the word "obedience," what does that bring to mind? You might initially think of obedience as being something unpleasant or burdensome or something that you *have* to do, but not willingly. Yet God equates obedience with love, joy and blessing.

We need look no further than the example of children to see how human nature often strains against the commands of a parent. Who hasn't seen a child react with reluctance (or even outright disobedience) when told to do something for "his or her own good"? Although most parents are acting in their children's best interest for their health and safety, children just naturally seem to strain at the reins. Parents set boundaries only to watch the child inch a toe over the line.

Wise parents lovingly discipline their recalcitrant children, for misbehavior must always be met with correction. We have all seen the results of a parent who does not correct a child's disobedience: an obnoxious little person that no one wants to be around and who often grows up to be an even more obnoxious adult.

Our loving heavenly Father wants the best for us and—even more than our own earthly parents—knows what our best interests are. Yet we, like little children, strain against His commands and fight any restrictions on our behavior or attitudes. Like the child who has had a boundary set, we inch our toe over the line He has drawn. And when we disobey, we will experience His discipline—just as a disobedient child receives correction from his or her loving parents.

In this week's study, we will find examples for and the consequences of obedience and disobedience. We will weigh the rewards of obedience against the cost of disobedience.

Day 1 · OUR ROLE MODELS

Father God, You are the perfect parent, setting loving standards and boundaries to protect me and help me mature. Thank You that I can trust that Your commands and will for my life are for my own good. Amen.

One of the best Old Testament examples of living in obedience to God's commands is found in the book of Daniel. In Daniel 1:5-17, Daniel and three other teenaged Israelite boys were captured when Babylon invaded Judah and conquered Jerusalem. They were then taken into King Nebuchadnezzar's palace to be trained to serve. These boys were chosen because of their intelligence and good looks, and they received a daily amount of food and wine from the king's own table. However, according to verse 8, what did Daniel and his three friends resolve to do when presented with the food and wine?

_____

_____

_____

What was the reaction of the official who was in charge of them? Of what was he afraid (vv. 9-10)?

_____

_____

_____

What test did Daniel and his three friends propose? What was the official's response to that proposal (vv. 12-14)?

_____

_____

_____

According to verse 17, what was the result of Daniel, Shadrach, Meshach and Abednego's 10-day test?

_____

_____

_____

Jesus, of course, is our ultimate role model for learning to obey God. The earliest example is found in Luke 2:41-52, when the 12-year-old Jesus and His family made their annual Passover pilgrimage to Jerusalem. According to Jesus, to whom was He first and foremost obedient (v. 49)?

_____

_____

_____

Even at this early age Jesus was intent on obeying His heavenly Father. Yet what does verse 51 say about His behavior toward His earthly parents after this incident?

_____

_____

_____

John 14:31 states that Jesus was obedient to His heavenly Father throughout His life here on this earth. In Matthew 26:36-45, we see that obedience was not easy even for Him. What does Jesus say in verse 38 that indicates just how much He was suffering?

_____

_____

_____

How many times did He pray to have this cup of suffering taken from Him? What does that tell you about the depth of His suffering?

_____

_____

_____

_____

Jesus knew what was going to take place over the next several hours of His life, and He agonized over what lay before Him. How does Philippians 2:6-8 describe what Jesus' obedience meant?

_____

_____

_____

In 1 John 3:21-22, what is the link between obedience and answered prayer?

_____

_____

_____

According to Luke 22:43, how did the Father answer these agonizing prayers of Jesus?

_____

_____

_____

According to Hebrews 5:8-9, what was God's ultimate purpose for Jesus' suffering and death?

_____

_____

_____

From Jesus' example, we can learn four important concepts about obedience: (1) we need to share our feelings and concerns honestly with God in prayer; (2) we must be willing to set aside our own desires if they are contrary to God's will for our lives; (3) we need always obey God even when it isn't always easy, because this will glorify Him; and (4) we can expect God to give us the strength to obey Him.

> *Father, thank You for the example that Jesus provides in learning how to be obedient even when it is difficult. Remind me that Your will has a greater purpose than what I desire. Amen.*

THE CALL TO OBEDIENCE

Day 2

> *O Lord, help me to remember that what You ask me to do is a part of Your greater plan. I want to express my love in obedience to You, but I am weak. Please give me Your strength to do Your will. Amen.*

Jesus' obedience to His Father's will cost Him everything, but it gained everything for all of us who trust Him with our lives and accept His gift of salvation and eternal life. Because of what Jesus did for us, He has a call on our lives—a call to obey the Father's will. This call to obedience requires a daily choice to do the will of God. What does Mark 8:34-36 say about the cost of following Jesus?

_____

_____

_____

_____

In 1 Samuel 15:1-21, there is a story concerning King Saul's disobedience. Quickly skim the verses. According to 1 Samuel 15:22, in what does the Lord delight?

_____

_____

_____

_____

Given the fact that we no longer give burnt offerings and sacrifices, to what could these actions be compared in the Church today?

_____

_____

_____

_____

What is the admonition found in Matthew 7:21? What is your reaction to that admonition?

_____

_____

_____

_____

Read 1 John 2:3-6 and record the point of each verse in your own words.

Verses	Point of the verse
1 John 2:3	
1 John 2:4	
1 John 2:5	
1 John 2:6	

What negative thoughts, if any, hold you back from obeying the Lord of all creation?

_____

_____

_____

_____

What is your greatest fear in fully obeying God? How can you turn that fear over to God in prayer?

_____

_____

_____

Many Christians obey reluctantly. What are some positive reasons for obeying the Lord?

_____

_____

_____

Dear Lord, when I am reluctant to obey You, remind me that You have only my best interests in mind. Help me see the joy of obedience as I seek to do Your will. Give me the desire to serve You with all my heart. Amen.

THE COST OF DISOBEDIENCE

Day 3

You are the almighty God of the universe, and yet You desire fellowship with me! That is awesome, yet I falter at complete obedience to Your commands. Help me to always desire obedience to You over my own will. Amen.

In yesterday's lesson, we read of Saul's rebellion against God. Review the admonition to Saul in 1 Samuel 15:22. What was the result of Saul's rebellion as recorded in verse 23?

_____

_____

_____

We do not read the full story in these few verses, but Saul had a long record of failing to obey the Lord, and God finally had to remove the kingship from him. God does give us second opportunities to repent from our willful disobedience, but there comes a time when there are no more chances. What does Deuteronomy 11:26-28 say about the choice between obedience and disobedience?

_____

_____

_____

Deuteronomy 28:15-19 lists some of the curses that would befall the Israelites if they did not obey God. Despite this warning, throughout the Old Testament we see a roller coaster of obedience and disobedience among the Israelites. But then, don't we do the same thing? What is the warning found in Ephesians 5:6-11 to those who disobey?

_____

_____

_____

What is the promise and warning in Isaiah 1:19-20?

_____

_____

_____

You may wonder why it seems that those who live in blatant disobedience to God seem to be blessed with prosperity while those who live obediently seem to not be so prosperous. Psalm 73 describes just those feelings. What does it say will eventually happen to the wicked (vv. 18-19,27)?

_____

_____

_____

Think about your own life for a moment. Are there any areas in which you need to repent so that you might be blessed?

_____

_____

_____

Heavenly Father, forgive me when I disobey You. Forgive me also when I obey reluctantly. Help me remember that You have promised blessing when I obey. Strengthen me to resist the temptations to disobey Your will. Amen.

THE REWARD OF OBEDIENCE

Day
4

Lord, You have shown me the cost of disobedience. Please help me to remember that when I must choose between obeying You or obeying my own desires. I ask for Your blessing as I study Your Word today. Amen.

Over the past few days, we have learned much about obedience and disobedience. Today we will discover the rewards and blessings of obedience. What is the warning and what is the promise found in Matthew 7:21?

_____

_____

_____

Our memory verse for this week comes from the "Upper Room discourse," when Jesus gave His final words of instruction to His disciples before His crucifixion. What does John 14:21 tell us that obedience proves?

_____

_____

_____

What is the common thread found in John 14:15,23,31; 15:9 10,14?

_____

_____

_____

What does the repetition of this common thread tell you about the importance of what Jesus was trying to teach His disciples?

_____

_____

_____

Dwelling in God's love is one of the rewards of obedience. What are the benefits of obedience as listed in the following verses?

Verse	Benefit of obedience
2 Chron. 31:20-21	
Luke 11:28	
2 Cor. 9:13	
1 John 2:17	
1 John 3:22	

Which of these benefits is most appealing to you when you are confronted with a situation where you must choose obedience over disobedience?

_____

_____

_____

What is one area in following the First Place 4 Health program in which you need to choose obedience? What would be the benefit if you were to choose obedience in this area?

_____

_____

_____

Lord Jesus, give me the strength and desire to answer "yes, Lord" when You call. God, You know my limits and weaknesses. You know every part of me. Help me to be obedient to Your will. Amen.

WHO'S IN CHARGE HERE?

Lord God, You have given me choices. Strengthen me to make the
choice of obedience over disobedience. Open my eyes and
mind to every opportunity to obey You. Amen.

We have learned over the past few days about being obedient to our heavenly Father's will. God has also set up a chain of authority for us here on earth. He has set up leaders in the home, workplace, community and national government for the purpose of living fruitful lives. What does Ephesians 6:1-2 tell us is our *first* most important earthly authority in our lives?

_____

_____

_____

What is the promised blessing for obedience in this relationship (v. 3)?

_____

_____

_____

Ephesians 6:5-8 and Colossians 3:22 describe another authority we must obey—our employers. According to these verses, with what kind of attitude should we be serving our employers?

_____

_____

_____

If you are in a position of leadership in the home, workplace or community, what should be your responsibility toward those under your authority (see Colossians 4:1)?

_____

_____

_____

According to Titus 3:1, to whom else should we be obedient?

_____

_____

_____

What are the reasons given in Romans 13:1-7 for submission to government authority?

_____

_____

_____

Is there ever a time when it is right to rebel against the authority God has placed over us? What do Acts 4:18-19 and 5:29 say about obedience to authority when it is counter to God's will?

_____

_____

_____

Is there someone in authority over you that you find hard to obey? Examine your attitude and ask God to strengthen you to have a servant heart toward that person. Remember that you can do all things through Christ who strengthens you (see Philippians 4:13). Write a prayer asking for Christ's strength to help you obey.

_____

_____

_____

_____

Thank You, sovereign Lord, that You have set a chain of authority over us to give us order in our lives. Sometimes it seems these authorities might be in the wrong, but help me remember that You have a plan and that ultimately all I need to do is be obedient to You. In Jesus' name and power, amen.

REFLECTION AND APPLICATION

*Father, it has been a hard week of facing my attitudes and behaviors.
Thank You for the promises You have given in Your Word for the rewards of
obeying You. Help me apply what I have learned this week. Amen.*

This week's memory verse gives clear instruction about obedience. Jesus
says that whoever hears His commands and obeys them is the one who
loves Him. Do you love Him? Are you keeping His commands? Are you
obeying His will? These may be hard questions to answer honestly. Saying
you love God is easy, but showing it by your obedience is more difficult.

Being obedient may be painful or uncomfortable at first, but the end results are the blessings you will receive as you see God's perfect will un-
folding in your life. Which of the blessings and benefits of living a life in
obedience to God's direction have you experienced? Which do you want
to experience?

_____

_____

_____

_____

What have you learned about obedience this week that you can apply to
each of the four aspects of your life?

Emotional

_____

_____

Spiritual

_____

_____

Mental

_____

_____

_____

Physical

_____

_____

_____

Are you ready to experience the joys and blessings of obedience to God?

> *Thank You, Lord, for what Your Word teaches and admonishes me. Thank You that You have given me Your Holy Spirit to help me know Your Word. Help me to listen to Your leading through the Holy Spirit. Create in me a new attitude when I am reluctant to obey. I love You, Lord. Amen.*

Day 7

REFLECTION AND APPLICATION

Praise the Lord, O my soul; all my inmost being, praise Your holy name. Let me not forget all Your benefits and Your forgiveness of my sins. You have redeemed my life from the pit and You crown me with love and compassion (see Psalm 103:1-4). Amen.

How can we obey God if we do not know Him and His teachings? Psalm 119:11 states, "I have hidden your word in my heart that I might not sin against you." The Scripture verses that you are encouraged to memorize each week are a beginning to hiding God's Word in your heart. As you read Scripture each week, look for other passages that speak to your needs and situations. Write them on a card and begin to learn those as well. As you learn to memorize God's Word, you will understand more of what He desires for you to do.

One of the problems of Scripture memory is remembering the reference. However, you can cement it in your mind if you repeat the reference before and after each time you say the verse. The music CD that accompanies this Bible study is also an excellent resource to help you memorize Scripture. Listen to it in your car or at home while you're doing chores or exercising. Through this practice, the Holy Spirit will be able to bring to your mind the truths you need in times of difficulty.

The following prayers from *Praying God's Word* will guide you in using the Scripture you memorize as your prayers.[1]

Oh Lord, in You my heart rejoices, for I trust Your Holy name.
May Your unfailing love rest upon me, O Lord, as I put my hope in You
(see Psalm 33:21-22).

Lord, I will praise You with an upright heart as I learn Your righteous
laws. I will obey Your decrees for I know You will not utterly forsake
me (see Psalm 119:7-8).

Lord God, I pray that Your love may abound in me more and more with
knowledge and depth of insight, so that I will know what is best and
that I may be pure and blameless; filled with the fruit of righteousness
that comes through Jesus Christ (see Philippians 1:9,11).

Heavenly Father, You have said that if I hear Your commands
and obey them, I show my love for You and that because You love me,
my Father will love me. Help me to be obedient and prove my love
for You (see John 14:21).

Note

1. Beth Moore, *Praying God's Word* (Nashville, TN: Broadman & Holman, 2000), pp. 254, 255, 321.

Group Prayer Requests

4 first place
health

Today's Date: _____

Name	Request

Results

_____
_____
_____
_____
_____
_____

there's no
excuse

Our society today excels at the art of making excuses for bad behavior. We have all heard politicians, CEOs and celebrities make excuses for their poor choices. There are even businesses now that will help you come up with good excuses, going so far as to provide alibis when needed! However, no matter how we try to wiggle out of the consequences of our unwise choices, God knows each of us from the inside out, and He will deal with our sin with hard consequences.

Why do we make excuses? It is often to avoid punishment for some of our decisions that were poorly made. Sometimes it is because we made choices on the spur of the moment without really thinking the situation through. At other times, we make wrong choices because we listened to bad advice from another person. However, whatever the reason, we need to remember that an excuse is a lie disguised as a reason. We cannot allow our sin nature to rule our behavior when temptation is placed in our path.

When God confronts us with our sin, our excuses are stripped away. There's no place to hide! In this week's study, we will examine how we can deal honestly with our excuses. We will also examine how real progress in life begins when we stop making excuses and start being honest with ourselves—and with God.

THE CHOICE

Lord, no one can hide from You. You know us inside out. I confess my folly in hiding from You. Reveal Yourself to me as I study Your Word today. Amen.

It may seem obvious, but let's see where this excuse making all began. When Adam and Eve were in the Garden of Eden, God gave them a choice—the most costly choice to ever be made. What was God's command in Genesis 2:16-17?

_____

_____

_____

What was the consequence of disobeying this command?

_____

_____

_____

Genesis 3 tells us what happened next. Read verses 1 through 5. How is the serpent described in verse 1?

_____

_____

_____

The serpent was Satan, our enemy, disguised as a beautiful creature. How did Satan's question create doubt about God's command in Genesis 2:17?

_____

_____

_____

What was Satan's deception in verse 4?

_____

_____

_____

How did Satan make the forbidden fruit seem appealing (v. 5)? To what in our human nature did he appeal?

_____

_____

_____

What are the three steps of Eve's temptation as described in the first part of verse 6?

_____

_____

_____

What was the result of her following these steps of temptation (v. 7)?

_____

_____

_____

God had given Adam and Eve all that they needed in the Garden of Eden, and yet they gave in to the devil's tempting lies and made the one wrong choice offered them. Why do you suppose God would give Adam and Eve this choice?

_____

_____

_____

We continue to have to make choices every day. Today, you have already made the choice to do your Bible study. What is another choice you know you will face today?

_____

_____

Conclude by writing a prayer in your journal, asking your Creator to help you make healthy choices for your wellbeing.

Father, I pray for Your strength to help me resist and flee Satan
when he tempts me with lies. Help me make the right choices in obedience
to Your will for my life. Amen.

Day 2 — HIDE AND SEEK

Father God, there is no hiding from Your presence. Open my eyes to
Your leading as I study Your Word today. Amen.

Yesterday, we read the story of Adam and Eve and learned how they made the wrong choice when they were confronted with Satan's lies. What was their response to their sin, as written in Genesis 3:7?

_____

_____

_____

Compare their "after" state in verse 7 with their "before" state in Genesis 2:25. Why were they suddenly ashamed of their bodies?

_____

_____

_____

Continue to read in Genesis 3:8-11. Why did Adam and Eve hide from the Lord God (v. 10)?

_____

_____

_____

In verse 9, "the LORD God called to the man, 'Where are you?'" Do you think God really did not know where Adam and Eve were? Why do you suppose He asked the question?

_____

_____

_____

What do Psalms 44:20-21; 139:1-12 and Proverbs 28:13 say about the folly of thinking we can hide from God?

_____

_____

_____

_____

No matter where we go we cannot hide from God, and we are only deluding ourselves if we think we can hide our sin from Him. What is the warning found in Isaiah 59:2?

_____

_____

_____

Are there times when you feel that God is not hearing you? What is it that you are trying to hide from your Creator, the One who knows you wholly inside and out? Write a prayer of confession in your prayer journal.

> *Heavenly Father, I ask forgiveness for trying to hide any secrets or sins from You. Help me to realize that You know all, and so hiding really serves no purpose. Help me to always be honest with You and with myself. Amen.*

EXCUSES, EXCUSES

Day 3

> *O Lord, my excuses are worthless before You. Teach me Your truth that I might deal with my sin. Amen.*

In Genesis 3:9, when the Lord God asked Adam, "Where are you?" what was Adam's response?

_____

_____

_____

_____

What was the Lord's response as recorded in verse 11?

_____

_____

_____

_____

Busted! God knew that Adam and Eve had disobeyed His command to not eat of the tree of the knowledge of good and evil, but He asked Adam anyway. What might be God's reason for asking this question, even though He already knew the answer?

_____

_____

_____

_____

Did Adam respond with confession of his transgression? What was his response (v. 12)?

_____

_____

_____

_____

How did Adam in a subtle way put the blame back on God?

_____

_____

_____

What are some excuses you have heard that blame God for people's own misbehavior?

_____

_____

_____

_____

Adam's excuse pointed the finger of blame directly at Eve. What was her response (v. 13)?

_____

_____

_____

Have you ever used the excuse "the devil made me do it"? Is that really true? Can the devil make you do anything you know you shouldn't? Satan's goal is to thwart God's plan for our lives and he will throw every temptation in his arsenal at us to bring us down—but we always have a choice. What is the promise found in 1 John 4:4?

_____

_____

_____

How does that encourage you when you are tempted to do wrong and then make excuses for your wrongdoing?

_____

_____

_____

> *Lord God, remind me again that I cannot hide anything from You.*
> *Thank You that I can rely on Your power to resist the temptations that*
> *come my way in life. Make me sensitive to the leading of Your Holy Spirit*
> *as I meet the challenges and temptations of this day. Amen.*

GUILTY AS CHARGED

Day 4

Father, I desire to walk in fellowship with You. Cleanse me from sin
so that there is no barrier to our fellowship today. Amen.

Adam and Eve tried to hide the shame of their sin by covering their exposed bodies with fig leaves (see Genesis 3:7), but nothing could hide their shame from a holy, omniscient God. Their guilt also kept them from wanting to spend time in fellowship with the Lord. Our guilt can do the same in our lives. Today, we will look at the biblical example of David and how guilt affected his life. David was a man who was declared as "a man after God's own heart" (Acts 13:22), and yet he succumbed to temptation and sinned. Read the account in 2 Samuel 11.

How did David's fall into sin parallel Eve's fall in Genesis 3:4?

_____

_____

_____

_____

What did David do to hide his guilt?

_____

_____

_____

Arranging the death of an innocent man is a pretty drastic measure to cover up sin. It compounded David's guilt, and it also involved others in his sinful behavior. In 2 Samuel 12, there is the account of Nathan the prophet confronting David about his sins. What was Nathan's message from God about the consequences of David's sin as found in verses 13-14?

_____

_____

_____

This week's memory verse is taken from one of David's psalms. Write it from memory here.

_____

_____

_____

_____

In Psalm 51, David honestly expressed his deepest emotions and contrition to God after Nathan confronted him with his sin. What was David's confession in verses 3 and 4?

_____

_____

_____

_____

What were his six urgent requests in verses 10-12?

1. _____
2. _____
3. _____
4. _____
5. _____
6. _____

According to verses 16-17, what sacrifice does God want from us?

_____

_____

_____

_____

_____

Although David confessed and repented from his sin, he would suffer the consequences of the sin as Nathan had warned him in 2 Samuel 12:11 and 14. Besides the death of his and Bathsheba's son, from that day on there was strife and rebellion among his children for the remainder of his life. God did extend his grace to David and Bathsheba and gave them a second son, Solomon, who became the king after David, and the Bible says that "the Lord loved him" (2 Samuel 12:24). Solomon would go on to build the Temple and acquire wisdom and wealth before he, too, would succumb to temptation. But that's a story for another day!

"Create in me a pure heart, O God, and renew a steadfast spirit within me. Restore to me the joy of my salvation and grant me a willing spirit to sustain me" (Psalm 51:10,12). Amen.

Day 5

OUR HOPE—GOD'S GRACE

O Lord, my Lord, You are my only hope for salvation and deliverance from my sin. Restore to me the joy of my salvation. Amen.

Psalm 32 is another of David's psalms. What is he describing in verses 3 and 4? How was the weight of his guilt affecting him?

_____

_____

_____

What happened when he acknowledged his sin, according to verse 5?

_____

_____

_____

What is the hope David gives in verses 1 and 2?

_____

_____

_____

Psalm 103 also speaks of God's forgiveness and His love for us. As you read Psalm 103, list at least five things that describe God and His gracious actions toward us.

1. _____

2. _____

3. _____

4. _____

5. _____

Which of these descriptions speak most eloquently to you today? Why?

_____

_____

_____

_____

John 3:16 is one of the most quoted Scriptures in the Bible. Can you repeat it from memory right now? What about the lesser-known verse that follows? What dimension does verse 17 add to the gift God gave us in Jesus?

_____

_____

_____

According to Titus 2:11-12, what does the grace of God teach us to do?

_____

_____

_____

How does Ephesians 2:8-9 describe God's grace? What does that mean to you personally?

_____

_____

_____

Jesus is God's gracious gift that He sent to save us and to set us free from the guilt and shame of sin. Have you accepted that gracious gift of Jesus Christ and committed your life to Him? If you haven't or are unsure about that step, please talk with your First Place 4 Health leader. If you have, you no longer need to hide from God!

> Lord, thank You for Your gracious gift of Jesus Christ, Your only
> begotten Son. Help me to live today buoyed by the reality
> of what You have done in my life. In the name of Jesus, amen.

REFLECTION AND APPLICATION

Search me, O God, and know my heart; test me and know my anxious thoughts. See if there is any offensive way in me and lead me in the way everlasting (see Psalm 139:23-24). Amen.

Isn't it ironic that the first choice in the world involved food? Of course, seeking nourishment is a basic need and essential for sustaining life, but in the Garden of Eden Adam and Eve had everything they needed to nourish their bodies. Yet they wanted the one thing they could not have. That is so like us—when we know we should not eat something, that is the one thing that occupies our thoughts.

What are one or two things you crave that you know you shouldn't have?

_____

_____

_____

_____

What excuses do people often give for the unhealthy choices they make?

_____

_____

_____

_____

What excuses do you think of for your own unhealthy choices?

_____

_____

_____

What are the consequences of your unhealthy choices?

_____

_____

_____

Let's call giving in to temptation and the excuses we use to cover them up what they are: sin! We need to be honest with ourselves and with God. God knows all you have ever done or will do. If you've made wrong choices in the past, confess them, and He will forgive you. If your choices have created tough consequences, accept them. Then God can begin to work to transform both you and your consequences into victorious living.

The following statements contain truths that will set you free. Check the statements you want to make part of your life as you leave the trap of excuses and pursue honesty.

- ❑ God knows everything about me and still loves me. I can be honest with Him.
- ❑ When I make wrong choices, I admit my sins and God forgives me.
- ❑ When my wrong choices create tough circumstances, I trust God to give me strength to work through them.
- ❑ I know I'm not perfect, but I am loved. God loves me just as I am. God loves me too much to allow me to stay where I am. God isn't finished with me yet.
- ❑ Satan may tempt me, but he cannot force me to make wrong choices. I can resist him. I choose to resist him through God's power.
- ❑ Sure, I've made some wrong choices in the past. God has forgiven my past. I've chosen to make Him first place in my life, and as a result of His power in my life, I have a great future.

When you recognize the fact that Satan will tempt you to make wrong choices, you can rely on the fact that God will help you to make right choices. Keep your eyes focused on Jesus and what He has promised to do for you. Satan will turn away each time you resist him, but he won't give up. Remember that "the one who is in you is greater than the one who is in the world" (1 John 4:4).

> *God, You know my sins; my guilt cannot be hidden from You.*
> *Forgive my weaknesses and restore my joy. Help me to remember*
> *that You are always greater than our enemy, Satan, and that You*
> *will give me the power to withstand temptation. Amen.*

REFLECTION AND APPLICATION

*Heavenly Father, thank You for forgiving my sins and making me a
new creation in Christ Jesus. Help me to memorize Your Word and learn
new ways of behaving and thinking. Amen.*

The key to making good decisions and right choices is to keep our eyes
focused on Jesus and the Word of God. As we've stated, one of the most
effective ways to do that is to memorize Scripture. When God's Word is
planted in our heart and soul, the Holy Spirit can bring His words to
mind when we need help. God's Word can also help us support others
who have choices to make. This is especially important for encouraging
and supporting each other in a First Place 4 Health group.

The memory verse for this week reminds us that God knows us inside and out. He knows our sins and our weaknesses. We cannot hide
our guilt from Him, just as Adam and Eve couldn't hide from God in
the Garden. And, also just like Adam and Eve, He gives us choices. We
make choices about what to wear, what to eat, how to respond to people,
what to do on the job, how to spend our time—the list is endless. The
question is whether we earnestly seek God's help in making those
choices. He is interested in everything we do, and He will give us the di-
rections we need for living our lives for Him—if we *ask*.

Oftentimes we can't undo the effects of our wrong choices and must
bear the consequences of our actions. Look at the results of Adam and
Eve's disobedience. However, like David, God will forgive us when we
come to Him with repentant hearts, and He will give us the strength and
wisdom to deal with our consequences.

God has given us His Word to help us make right choices. When you
pray, use God's Word sincerely and with true repentance, meaning what
you say. Avoid merely saying the words, but understand and mean the
words with all your heart. Pray sincerely, believing His Word and listening for His direction as you pray this week.

Remember the words of Jesus: "Therefore I tell you, whatever you
ask for in prayer, believe that you have received it, and it will be yours"

(Mark 11:24). Claim God's promises in your prayer time and use His Word as you pray.

Lord, keep me from making excuses. Help me to serve only You. For You have promised to always be with me, to hold me by my right hand, to guide me with Your counsel and then to take me to glory (see Psalm 73:23-24).

Merciful God, hear my prayer. I confess my sin to You for You have promised to forgive my wickedness and remember my sins no more (see Jeremiah 31:34).

Heavenly Father, forgive my sin for You know my folly, and my guilt cannot be hidden from You (see Psalm 69:5). Amen.

Group Prayer Requests

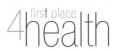

Today's Date: _____

Name	Request

Results

_____

_____

_____

_____

_____

_____

don't
tempt me!

SCRIPTURE MEMORY VERSE
*No temptation has seized you except what is common to man.
And God is faithful; he will not let you be tempted beyond
what you can bear. But when you are tempted, he will also
provide a way out so that you can stand up under it.*
1 CORINTHIANS 10:13

As we read last week, temptation has been with us since the fall of mankind in the Garden of Eden when Satan deceived Adam and Eve into eating the one thing the Lord had told them not to eat—the fruit of the tree of the knowledge of good and evil. Ever since that time, mankind has struggled with the deception of the devil whose main purpose has been to thwart God's plan for the world.

The Bible is filled with stories of many people who walked in close fellowship with the Lord and how they also succumbed to temptation. None of us are exempt from the pull of our own fleshly desires and the devil's schemes to draw us away from the Lord. However, there is hope in our faithful heavenly Father, who loves us so much that He gave His only Son to this world and to us to save us from our sins. That Son had to endure temptation just as we did, but He was able to withstand it and not sin.

In this week's study, we will explore more about temptation and how to withstand its wiles. Once again, Jesus is our role model as we learn to stand up under the weight of temptation.

TYPES OF TEMPTATION

O Lord, help me to learn more about You from Your Word today.
Show me how to resist temptation. Amen.

In last week's lesson, we saw the results of giving in to temptation in Genesis 3 when Adam and Eve willfully disobeyed God's command to not eat of the tree of the knowledge of good and evil. We saw that there is a descent from temptation into sin. Notice the three basic categories of temptation as found in 1 John 2:16: "For all that is in the world, the [1] lust of the flesh and the [2] lust of the eyes and the [3] boastful pride of life, is not from the Father, but is from the world" (1 John 2:16, *NASB*).

Match the temptation in Genesis 3:6 with those listed in 1 John 2:16.

Genesis 3:6	1 John 2:16
	The lust of the flesh
	The lust of the eyes
	The boastful pride of life

How does James 1:14-15 describe the descent from temptation to sin? What does sin give birth to?

_____

_____

_____

How can knowing the types of temptation help us when we feel the pull to give in to the temptations we encounter?

_____

_____

_____

In what ways are you most tempted?

_____

_____

_____

What part of the First Place 4 Health program are you most tempted to not participate in? What would happen if you resisted that temptation and participated wholeheartedly?

_____

_____

_____

Reread this week's memory verse. How can this verse give you courage and strength to resist the temptations you face?

_____

_____

_____

Thank You, Father God, that You have promised to help me when I am tempted. Help me to discern those things that tempt me and give me the strength to stand against their pull. Amen.

COMMON TO MAN

Day 2

Lord, help me understand Your Word as I study today. Show me the lessons that You have specifically for me. Keep my mind and heart open to Your instruction. Amen.

Our memory verse states that *everyone* is tempted to follow their fleshly desires. Even Jesus was tempted, as we will see in Matthew 4. What took place just before Jesus' temptation, as recorded in Matthew 3:13-17?

_____

_____

_____

This incident was a spiritual high point for the beginning of Jesus' ministry. What happened next according to Matthew 4:1? What warning do you see in the close relationship of the spiritual high and the temptation that came afterward?

_____

_____

_____

_____

Read Matthew 4:1-10. Notice that this passage states that Jesus had been fasting for 40 days and 40 nights. Notice also that the first temptation was focused on Jesus' most immediate and most basic need: food. What does this tell you about the devil's tactics?

_____

_____

_____

_____

What weapon did Jesus use against Satan in each of these temptations?

_____

_____

_____

Read Luke 4:1-12. What were the three temptations, and how do they compare to the passage in 1 John 2:16 that we read yesterday?

Luke 4:1-12	1 John 2:16
	The lust of the flesh
	The lust of the eyes
	The boastful pride of life

Some might point out that because Jesus was also divine, it was easy for Him to resist the devil's schemes to thwart God's purpose. How does Hebrews 2:17-18 refute that theory?

_____

_____

_____

Jesus faithfully resisted temptation without sinning. Because He has done it, so can we! What hope do you find in Hebrews 2:18 that can help you this week as you meet with the temptations you will encounter?

_____

_____

_____

Lord, thank You that Jesus set such a shining example of how to resist. Bring to mind Your Word, the sword of the Spirit, to help me in times of weakness.

GOD IS FAITHFUL

Day 3

O righteous Lord, thank You that You are faithful to Your promises. Teach me more about Your faithfulness as I study Your Word today. Amen.

Yesterday, we explored the account of Jesus' temptation in the desert after His baptism. In that study, we pointed out that Jesus was tempted as we are, but He did not sin. What does Luke 4:13 add to the story that was not in the Matthew account of the temptation of Jesus?

_____

_____

_____

How does this addition relate to the comfort found in Hebrews 4:15-16?

_____

_____

_____

What do the following verses say about God?

Deuteronomy 7:9

_____

_____

_____

_____

1 Corinthians 1:9

_____

_____

_____

_____

1 Thessalonians 5:23-24

_____

_____

_____

_____

2 Thessalonians 3:3

_____

_____

_____

_____

One of the central principles of the Christian life is God's faithfulness. We can affirm His faithfulness intellectually, but it is through our experiences with Him that we will come to know God's faithfulness personally and emotionally. What is the promise in Psalm 73:26?

_____

_____

_____

Have you experienced God's faithfulness in dealing with temptation? What was the result?

_____

_____

_____

We learned yesterday that Jesus was able to withstand temptation after fasting for 40 days and nights. What does Matthew 4:11 say happened after the devil left Jesus alone? How could that encourage you when you are tempted and struggling to resist?

_____

_____

_____

_____

_____

Philippians 4:13 states, "For I can do everything with the help of Christ who gives me the strength I need" (*NLT*). Do you believe that? Look at all that He has done for you already. Can you trust Him to do what He has promised?

> *I praise You, O God, for You are faithful to keep all Your promises. Let me not forget that You are the strength of my heart and my portion forever. I need nothing else but You, O Lord. Amen.*

WHAT YOU CAN BEAR

Day 4

> *O holy God, help me to understand Your teaching and apply it to my circumstances today. Amen.*

God never promised that we would not be tempted or that temptations would be easy for us to resist. He has, however, set limits on the degree to which we can be tempted. As Paul states in this week's Memory Verse,

He will not let us be tempted beyond what we can bear. God knows what level of temptation we *are able to* bear, and He has given us the resources we need to resist.

Did you notice the first few words of this verse: "No temptation has *seized* you" (emphasis added)? Have you ever felt like temptation has *seized* you—like you had no control over the situation? Some might excuse themselves by saying, "I couldn't help myself." What are some other excuses you have seen people use when they have given in to temptation?

_____

_____

_____

What does James 1:14 say about such excuses? What phrase in this verse is similar to being "seized" by temptation?

_____

_____

_____

Being tempted is a trial or a test of our maturity in Christ. What is the purpose of testing according to James 1:2-4?

_____

_____

_____

What does James 1:12 promise when we persevere under trial?

_____

_____

_____

The "crown of life" here refers to the type of crown, or wreath, that would have been given to a victorious athlete or military leader. When we resist temptation, it is a victory in our spiritual growth. Have you experienced that sense of victory when you have successfully resisted a temptation? Describe your experience.

_____

_____

_____

God has promised us the strength we need to resist temptation. In Ephesians 3:14-21, Paul wrote a prayer for the church. Read the passage, and then write verses 16-17 as a prayer for yourself.

_____

_____

_____

Consider the temptations Christ endured for our salvation. Recall His temptations in the desert. Remember His agony in the Garden of Gethsemane when He prayed to have the cup taken from Him. What a tremendous temptation it must have been for Him to simply walk away from what He would endure for our sakes! But because Jesus did not walk away from the path set before Him, we have the power of His Holy Spirit dwelling in us to resist any temptation that God allows. We can bear it with His love and strength.

> *Almighty God, You are able to do immeasurably more than all I can ask or imagine, according to Your power that is at work within me. Thank You that I will not be tempted beyond what I can bear. Amen.*

THE WAY OUT

Day
5

> *Omnipotent Father, to You be the glory in the Church and in Christ Jesus throughout all generations, for ever and ever (see Ephesians 3:21). Amen.*

In 1 Corinthians 10:13, Paul warns that temptation *will* come to us. Notice that he says "*when* you are tempted" rather than "*if* you are tempted."

What is the promise given at the end of the verse?

_____

_____

_____

We know that God has provided a way out, but we must look for that escape route. We must make the choice to resist temptation on a daily basis.
What does James 4:7 instruct us to do that can also relate to temptation?

_____

_____

_____

In 1 Peter 5:8-9, how is the devil described? What is he looking for?

_____

_____

_____

What is the admonition found in the first part of verse 8?

_____

_____

_____

There is another admonition in verse 9. What words in 1 Peter 5:9 are repeated in Ephesians 6:11,13-14?

_____

_____

_____

Do you understand the command to resist and to stand against the
devil? We are not to be passive in resisting temptation but are to stand
firmly. God has given us all we need, and He backs us up with His
strength and mighty power (see Ephesians 6:10). As we studied earlier,
our greatest weapon against temptation is God's Word. How are you do-

ing in building your arsenal of Scripture verses? Have you had a recent experience of using God's Word to resist temptation? If so, describe it.

_____

_____

_____

_____

Another way to prepare to fight temptation is to recognize times when temptation strikes. Maybe there are certain times of the year that you find especially difficult to stick to your Live It plan, your exercise routine or your Bible study. That might be a vacation time, when busyness takes over and overindulgence is expected (and even encouraged). Or maybe there is a time of day that you are more prone to snack on junk food. What are the times that you find you are most vulnerable to temptation?

_____

_____

_____

_____

What can you plan to do to resist this temptation? For instance, if there is a time of day when you are more tempted to grab that candy bar, prepare yourself with a healthy alternative. It might be having a piece of fruit available, or it might be to take a walk instead. What will be your plan of attack?

_____

_____

_____

_____

Lord, You have promised a way out of temptation when I need it.
Please help me to recognize Your escape plan, and give me the
strength to take that exit route. Thank You that You have given
me all I need to live a victorious life in Christ Jesus. Amen.

REFLECTION AND APPLICATION

Thank You, O God, that You have given me the power to withstand temptation. Help me to memorize Your Word to build my arsenal and to stand firm against the devil's schemes. Amen.

God has given us His armor to protect us from the "flaming arrows of the evil one" (Ephesians 6:16). In Ephesians 6:18, Paul describes another tactic we can use against our enemy: prayer. Do you pray daily—even hourly or minute by minute—for God's help in resisting the temptations that come your way? Just as important, do you pray regularly for your First Place 4 Health group members?

One of the greatest gifts we can give to others is our earnest prayer for their needs. Each week at your weekly meeting, you and your group members share prayer requests. Be diligent in praying for these requests and ask God to strengthen others as they encounter the temptations along their path to healthy, balanced living. Honestly share your own struggles and triumphs in your journey. It will encourage others.

What is one thing your fellow group members can pray for you during this coming week? (Be sure to list this prayer request on the Group Prayer Requests form at the end of this session.)

_____

_____

_____

What have you learned this week that has been especially helpful in resisting temptation? How can you share that lesson with others?

_____

_____

_____

Unfortunately, there will be times when you will give in to temptation no matter how hard you try to resist. You may be in a weakened state due to fatigue or stress, or you might simply be feeling rebellious. At some point, you will become vulnerable and give in. And when you give in, feelings of defeat, worthlessness or depression can set in as you try to cope with your failure to be obedient. Hopefully, as you practice the things we've learned this week, the failures will be fewer and fewer—but understand that they *will* happen, as we are humans living in a fallen world.

When you do give in to temptation, you have one recourse: fall at the foot of God's throne in repentance. He has promised to forgive us and cleanse us from all unrighteousness (see 1 John 1:9). When you get up again, you will have a new beginning and a fresh start. So do not give up. God is with you all the way. Your heavenly Father wants you to be victorious in this battle against temptation!

Lord, thank You for providing a way out of sin for me. Shed Your light on the path ahead so that I will recognize the temptations as they come. Strengthen me in using the sword of the Spirit, Your Word. Amen.

REFLECTION AND APPLICATION

Day 7

Almighty God, You are faithful to all Your promises. You have promised to be with me as I walk this troubled world. Thank You for Your lovingkindness toward me. Amen.

The most serious consequence of giving in to temptation is that each unchecked sin can lead to strongholds that will take over your life and destroy your relationships with the Lord and others. Strongholds are those repeated sins that replace God's position and influence in your life. Read 2 Corinthians 10:3-5 to refresh your memory about the damage of strongholds.

God can and will forgive you and release you from these strongholds. However, once God has forgiven you and you have put those temptations out of your life, Satan will continue to bring them up and entice you into his ways once again. You must always be self-controlled and alert for those temptations he will use to try to lure you back into your former strongholds (see 1 Peter 5:8-9). God's Word becomes the exit, the way out for you.

The key to resisting temptation is the same as you would use in making choices: keep your eyes focused on Jesus. Let your words and your thoughts be centered on Him. Again, reading God's Word daily and committing it to memory will assure that you will have His words ready to help you in any situation. Jesus battled Satan with God's truth, and you will have to do the same. Each verse you memorize will provide another weapon in your arsenal in the battle against temptation.

God is committed to building your character and transforming you into the image of Christ. He wants you to be mature and complete, not lacking in anything. But that transformation won't be quick or easy. You will face trials and temptations, and you will stumble and fall along the way. But remember God's promise in Deuteronomy 30:11: He will not command you to do anything that is too difficult or beyond your reach. Remind yourself of this as you face the trials and temptations that come into your life.

Pray today for God's protection in times of temptation. Put on His whole armor, arm yourself with the sword of the Spirit, and stand fast in your faith.

Father God, Your Word says I am to love the Lord and hate evil, for You will guard the life of Your faithful servant and deliver me from the hand of the wicked. Deliver me, O God, from the lies of Satan (see Psalm 97:10).

Merciful God, You are my hiding place. You will protect me from trouble and surround me with songs of deliverance (see Psalm 32:7).

Father, You taught us to pray, asking to not yield to temptation and to be delivered from evil, for Yours is the kingdom and the power and the glory forever. Deliver me from the evil one and all his lies so I may live with You eternally (see Matthew 6:13).

Mighty God, You instructed me not to love the world or the things in the world, for if I love the world, the love of the Father is not in me. Everything that tempts me from the world—the lust of the flesh, the lust of the eyes and the pride of life—is not of You, O Father. Help me to love You and only You, and dwell in me so that I may not sin (see 1 John 2:15-16).

Father God, help me to get rid of all immoral filth and the evil that is so prevalent, and help me to humbly accept the Word planted in me which can save me (see James 1:21).

Faithful heavenly Father, I know Your Word and trust You because You have told me that temptation is common to all people and that You will not allow me to be tempted with anything I cannot bear. I claim Your promise of provision for a way out so that I can stand firm and strong against any temptation (see 1 Corinthians 10:13).

Group Prayer Requests

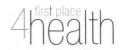

Today's Date: _____

Name	Request

Results

_____

_____

_____

_____

_____

_____

a spiritual
feast

SCRIPTURE MEMORY VERSE
*Man does not live on bread alone, but on
every word that comes from the mouth of God.*
MATTHEW 4:4

This week's lesson might be a touchy topic for those of us who struggle with keeping our weight under control. We will be discussing food—spiritual food, that is! Hopefully, the study will help focus on eternal food that only Jesus offers, not the attraction of temporal food.

When you experience physical hunger or thirst, what thoughts fill your mind? Most likely it is thoughts of what you want to eat, what you crave. That is the kind of attitude we should have about the spiritual food God offers in His Word. Do you crave the time you spend in studying the Bible? Do you look forward to the time you spend in prayer, in fellowship with the Lord? Do you eagerly attend church each Sunday? In this week's lesson, we will look at ways to develop that craving for the Lord in our heart, soul, mind and spirit.

HUNGRY? THIRSTY?

Day
1

O Lord my God, make me hunger for the spiritual food You offer
Teach me from Your Word today. Amen.

This week's memory verse may seem familiar to you, as we just studied the temptation of Jesus last week. The verse comes from Jesus' 40 days in the desert when Satan was tempting Him to turn the stones to bread. Can you imagine what a temptation that must have been after 40 days of fasting? Yet Jesus was so focused on obedience to His Father that He resisted the temptation that Satan laid out before Him.

What is the longest you have ever had to go without food? Perhaps it was for a medical test or for surgery, or perhaps you have tried fasting for spiritual purposes. What was foremost in your mind during this experience?

_____

_____

_____

Have you ever been really thirsty? What were your feelings and thoughts during that experience?

_____

_____

_____

_____

Read the Beatitudes in Matthew 5:1-10. The word "blessed" can also mean "happy." What does Matthew 5:6 say we should seek, and with what kind of intensity?

_____

_____

_____

What is the reward for this seeking?

_____

_____

_____

"Righteousness" means being in right fellowship with God. If you hunger and thirst for your time in fellowship with God, you will be satisfied. Do you have this kind of intense desire for seeking righteousness? Why or why not?

_____

_____

_____

In Romans 1:17, Paul states what the basis of our righteousness should be before God. What is that basis?

_____

_____

_____

Until our relationship with God is right, our lives won't be right. We each have a fundamental spiritual need for God, and we can't experience lasting satisfaction in our lives until we establish our relationship with God through Jesus Christ. Through faith, however, we can have that right standing with God because Jesus Christ died for us. If God had not paid for our sins on the cross, we could never experience His love. Our sin would demand God's judgment and would keep us separated from Him. Ephesians 2:4-10 contains wonderful truth about salvation. What does this passage tell us about the basis of our relationship with God?

_____

_____

_____

Check the following statements that are true about you. If you cannot check every box, talk with your pastor, your First Place 4 Health leader or a Christian friend about your uncertainty

- ❑ I have begun a relationship with Jesus Christ.
- ❑ I am now righteous in God's eyes because of my faith in Christ.
- ❑ I have right standing with God because of Jesus' death on the cross.
- ❑ I am sure I am a Christian.

Lord, help me to grow in my relationship with You. Thank You for loving me and for sending the Holy Spirit to live in me. Thank You for forgiving my sins. Guide me in all that I do as I work toward my goal. Amen.

Day
2

THE BREAD OF LIFE

Heavenly Father, thank You for Your Word that encourages, comforts, teaches and admonishes me to live a Christlike life. Open my heart, mind, soul and spirit to Your truth today. Amen.

Bread has been the main source of sustenance for people throughout history. It is mentioned more than 300 times in both the Old and New Testaments, often with a spiritual connection. When Jesus put off the devil's temptation by stating, "Man does not live on bread alone, but on every word that comes from the mouth of God" (Matthew 4:4), He was repeating the words found in Deuteronomy 8:3. What added dimension does this Scripture add to this week's memory verse?

_____

_____

_____

_____

In John 6:1-13, we find the story of Jesus feeding the 5,000. What was the reaction of the people as recorded in verses 14-15? What did Jesus do?

_____

_____

_____

The very next day, the people came looking for Jesus (vv. 24-25). What was their focus, and how did Jesus rebuke them (vv. 26-27)?

_____

_____

_____

As you read verses 26-35, note the statements that Jesus made about bread and the spiritual applications for these truths. How did Jesus describe Himself in John 6:35? What is the promise in this verse?

_____

_____

_____

In John 6:49-51, Jesus compares Himself with the manna that God gave to the Jews in the desert. What is the distinction that Jesus made between manna and Himself?

_____

_____

_____

How can these word pictures of Jesus as the "bread of life" and "the bread come down from heaven" encourage you as you follow the First Place 4 Health program?

_____

_____

_____

> *Heavenly Father, thank You for Your provision of Jesus as the "bread of life" and the "bread that came down from heaven" to feed me for all eternity. May I fill up on Your bread today that I might not hunger for worldly things that do not satisfy. Amen.*

THE ENTREE

Day 3

> *Thank You, Father, for sending our bread of life, Jesus, to save us from sin and give us food that will not leave us hungry or thirsty. Amen.*

Jesus is our bread of life, and God's Word, the Bible, is also part of the feast of spiritual food that God has provided for us. The Old Testament prophet Ezekiel received a vision from God that involved a literal feasting on spiritual food. The experience is described in Ezekiel 3:1-3. What was Ezekiel asked to do?

_____

_____

_____

What does this word picture suggest to you? How can someone eat God's Word?

_____

_____

_____

How did Ezekiel describe the taste of God's Word in verse 3?

_____

_____

_____

In Psalm 119:103, how is God's Word described?

_____

_____

_____

How did Jeremiah describe the experience of eating God's Word in Jeremiah 15:16?

_____

_____

_____

What has been your experience in consuming God's Word? Is it your joy and your heart's delight?

_____

_____

_____

Each of the following verses instructs us in how to learn God's Word. As you read each verse, summarize in a word or short phrase what it says about dealing with the Word, and then list at least one specific way you can put this into practice.

Verse	Summary	Application
Neh. 8:8-10		
Ps. 1:2		
Ps. 119:11		
Rom. 10:17		
2 Tim. 2:15		
2 Tim. 3:16		
Jas. 1:22		
Rev. 1:3		

Why is doing as these verses suggest so important to your spiritual growth as a Christian?

_____

_____

_____

_____

What is one action you will take in partaking of God's Word?

_____

_____

_____

_____

> *Father God, Your words are sweeter than honey to my mouth and to my soul. Help me to eat of it and be filled daily. Show me how to act on what I read and hear from Your Word. Amen.*

Day 4 — WHAT'S TO DRINK?

Lord, open my eyes today that I may see the many opportunities for witnessing and sharing Your living water with others. Amen.

The Jews and the Samaritans had an intense hatred for one another. They disagreed on how and where to worship God. Samaria was the region that lay between Galilee and Judea, but the Jews would avoid traveling through Samaria whenever possible. But in John 4:4, Jesus and His disciples traveled through Samaria on the way back to Galilee from Judea. Read Jesus' encounter with the woman in the Samaritan village of Sychar in John 4:4-15. Where had the disciples gone (v. 8)?

_____

_____

_____

The sixth hour was about noon. It was unusual for the village women to draw their water at that time, so Jesus and the woman were alone at the well. What was Jesus' simple request, and what was the woman's answer (vv. 7-9)?

_____

_____

_____

How does Jesus compare the well water with the living water He offered (vv. 13-14)?

_____

_____

_____

Notice the phrase "a spring of water welling up to eternal life." The phrase has the connotation of gushing forth. Can you picture it in your mind? What was the woman's response when she heard this phrase (v. 15)?

_____

_____

_____

Continue reading in John 4:16-38. Jesus then confronted the woman about her sin. What was her declaration about Jesus in verse 19? Why did she make this connection?

_____

_____

_____

When the woman spoke of the coming Messiah, what was Jesus' response (v. 26)? What was her reaction to His response (vv. 28-29)?

_____

_____

_____

When the disciples returned, they urged Jesus to eat. His response was, "I have food to eat that you know nothing about" (John 4:32). Unfortunately, the disciples missed Jesus' intended meaning. What was Jesus actually saying about the food He had to offer?

_____

_____

_____

Jesus taught the disciples that doing the Father's work was like eating spiritual food. It satisfied Him so fully that physical food was less important to Him. The disciples were so focused on taking care of their physical needs that they were missing the spiritual opportunities around them. According to John 4:39-42, what was the result of Jesus giving the Samaritan woman living water?

_____

_____

_____

Can you imagine how that village was transformed? Jesus offered living water and reaped a spiritual bumper crop. The disciples were focused on physical needs and would have missed the spiritual harvest had Jesus not shown them the difference. In your own words, describe the truth found in Isaiah 55:1-2.

_____

_____

_____

_____

What does 1 Peter 2:2 say about milk in relation to spiritual growth?

_____

_____

_____

Look up 1 Corinthians 3:1-2 and Hebrews 5:11-14. How do these passages compare milk to solid food?

_____

_____

_____

We are admonished to crave spiritual milk as infants do, but then we must grow up and eat the solid food of deeper learning, digging into

God's Word, becoming more mature in our faith. Where are you on this journey? Place an *X* on the line to show your position.

_____

Milk   Solid Food

Heavenly Father, fill me with the living water of eternal life that it might well up into the lives of others. Move me from craving spiritual milk to partaking of the solid food of Your truth. Amen.

BON APPÉTIT!   Day 5

Almighty God, You have given a feast in Your Word. Show me what I need to fill up on today. Amen.

This week, we have been studying about spiritual food and drink. Hopefully, this has whetted your spiritual appetite for more of God's Word— and not your physical appetite! Today, we will discuss the byproduct of satisfying our spiritual hunger: contentment.

In 2 Corinthians 11:23-33, Paul lists some of the hardships he endured for the work of taking the gospel to the world. Scan the passage and list a few of the hardships he endured.

_____

_____

_____

_____

In Philippians 4:11-12, Paul speaks of contentment despite all of his sufferings. Summarize his statement.

_____

_____

_____

_____

What does Philippians 4:19 reveal about the secret to contentment?

_____

_____

_____

How does Psalm 34:8-10 relate to our spiritual food theme this week?
What is the result of "tasting" the Lord?

_____

_____

_____

What does Psalm 90:14 ask of God?

_____

_____

_____

What is the response to that love? Can you honestly say that it is your
response? Why or why not?

_____

_____

_____

In 1 Timothy 6:6, Paul states, "Godliness with contentment is great gain."
How have you seen that take place in your life or in the lives of others?

_____

_____

_____

_____

What does Hebrews 13:5 say about the secret to contentment?

_____

_____

_____

Have you experienced the contentment that comes from seeking spiritual food and living water that Jesus offers? Examine your life and see where you need more spiritual sustenance to bring true contentment. Invite Jesus in (see Revelation 3:20); sit down with Him and have a spiritual feast. Write in your prayer journal about your experience. Bon appétit! Enjoy the meal!

Lord, I know that only You can satisfy my emotional hunger. Become the bread of life in my life today. Jesus, I want to open the door for You to enter into my life completely. I invite You to come in and take total control of my life.

REFLECTION AND APPLICATION

Day
6

Lord Jesus, You are the bread of life and giver of living water. When I feast on Your provisions, I am filled to overflowing. Amen.

We have spent the past week learning about the satisfaction that only spiritual food and drink can bring to our body, spirit, mind and emotions. We have also discussed the importance of looking to God to satisfy our hunger. Too many people continue to hope that food, alcohol, drugs, sex or other temptations will satisfy that inner hunger.

In Galatians 5:19-21, Paul lists a number of sinful acts and warns that those who live sinful lives cannot inherit the kingdom of God. While you may not be tempted by many of these sins, remember that no one is immune from all of them—and that if you think you are immune, you may be being deceived by Satan into thinking you are okay and don't need to worry. It is in those instances that you will be tempted to let your guard down, which will give Satan his opportunity.

Look at some of the sins listed in verse 20: jealousy, anger, selfishness, selfish ambition, discord and dissension. Be careful that none of these emotional feelings or actions causes you to stumble. Also notice that this is not an all-inclusive list, because Paul adds the phrase "and the like" at the end of the passage. What Paul is saying is that there are other things that might trip you up as well.

Can you handle one more allusion to food? There is another kind of spiritual food that the Bible teaches about: the fruit of the Spirit. Read about it in Galatians 5:22-23. The fruit of the Spirit is:

Love	Joy	Peace
Patience	Kindness	Goodness
Faithfulness	Gentleness	Self-Control

Notice that although this list includes nine items, Paul refers to the group in the singular—as the *fruit* of the Spirit. That means that when the Holy Spirit is dwelling in us, we should exhibit *all* of these characteristics, not just some of them. Think about this in your own life. Which of the traits on this list do you feel that you are exhibiting already? Which need some work? Which are not there at all? Spend some time in your prayer journal discussing the fruit of the Spirit in your life.

Only in Christ can you find true satisfaction in life. Through Him you will find the strength to meet the demands of everyday living. The good news is that when you focus on Him and confess your sins to Him, the fruit of the Spirit will mature in your life.

Father God, I confess the sins that keep me from experiencing true contentment. I pray for the fruit of the Spirit—love, joy, peace, patience, kindness, goodness, faithfulness, gentleness and self-control—to become more evident in my life. Amen.

Day 7

REFLECTION AND APPLICATION

O Lord, help me to apply Your instruction to my life so that the fruit of Your Holy Spirit will be evident and that my actions would glorify You. Amen.

This week's memory verse should remind you that God provides what you need daily through His Word. When physical desires begin to take over control, you can turn to the Bible for the comfort and spiritual food that will help you resist the physical desires that are destructive to the balance in your life. When you have Scripture memorized, you have His Word at your disposal anytime and anywhere.

There are still places in many countries around the world where few people have access to the Bible in print. Can you imagine how precious God's Word is to those who cannot own their own copy? They must learn the Word from one another, relying on memorizing Scripture. Could you quote and then write down enough verses to fill a book? What a challenge!

Remember that God's Word is the sword of the Spirit—your offensive weapon against the enemy. Repeat the memory verses often, and remember to say the reference before and after each repetition. Each time you use the verse, God will plant this Scripture more firmly in your mind and heart, and through confidence in God's provision, you will be better able to resist the temptations that come into your life.

Father, help me to be both filled and hungry, to both abound and suffer need because I know that true contentment comes only from You. I can do all things through Jesus, Your Son, who strengthens me (see Philippians 4:12-13).

Merciful God, it is only because of Your great love for me and the richness of Your mercy that I was made alive in Christ even when I was dead in sin. Your grace has saved me (see Ephesians 2:4-5).

Heavenly Father, feed me with Your Word, for You have said that man does not live on bread alone, but on every word that comes from the mouth of God (see Matthew 4:4). Amen.

Group Prayer Requests

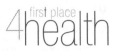

Today's Date: _____

Name	Request

Results

_____

_____

_____

_____

_____

_____

a new
you

SCRIPTURE MEMORY VERSE

*Do not conform any longer to the pattern of this world,
but be transformed by the renewing of your mind.
Then you will be able to test and approve what
God's will is—his good, pleasing and perfect will.*

ROMANS 12:2

You've heard all of the promises: A new you in 90 . . . 60 . . . 30 . . . even 14 days! Whether it's weight loss, body toning, plastic surgery or teeth whitening, the world promises big but delivers little. The truth is that there is only one way to have a new you, and that is through the transformation that occurs when you accept Jesus Christ as Savior and Lord of your life.

The process of transformation began the moment you accepted Jesus into your life and will continue until that glorious day when you are taken up to heaven to be with Him forever. As Paul describes in Ephesians 4:22-24, this spiritual journey requires you to take off the "old" self and put on the "new" self. God will transform you into a new creation as He does His good work in you moment by moment and day by day over the course of a lifetime. In theological terms, this lifelong process is called "sanctification."

As we work our way through this week's Scripture memory verse, we will learn what it means to be truly transformed by the Lord Jesus Christ dwelling within us.

THE PATTERN OF THIS WORLD

Heavenly Father, teach me Your Word so that my mind may be renewed and I no longer want to conform to this world. Amen.

In Matthew 16:26, Jesus posed this question: "What good will it be for a man if he gains the whole world, yet forfeits his soul? Or what can a man give in exchange for his soul?" As we begin to consider the influence that the forces of this world have on us, what warning does this provide to us?

_____

_____

_____

According to 1 John 5:19, "the whole world is under the control of the evil one." At first, this might seem surprising. Isn't God the sovereign ruler of everything? However, in John 14:30, we see that Jesus describes the devil as "the prince of this world." What kinds of power does a prince usually have in an earthly kingdom? Who usually gives a prince his power?

_____

_____

_____

From history, we know that princes often try to usurp a king's power and take over the kingdom. As you read the following verses, match what each passage says about the pattern of this world:

____ John 15:18-19	a. A friend of the world is an enemy of God.
____ 1 Corinthians 3:19	b. Destined for destruction, ruled by appetites; relishing shameful things.
____ Philippians 3:18-19	c. There are many false prophets in the world.
____ James 4:4	d. The world hates Jesus' followers.
____ 1 John 2:16	e. The world's wisdom is foolishness compared to God's.
____ 1 John 4:1	f. The world encourages the lust of the flesh, the lust of the eyes and the boastful pride of life.

How is the devil described in John 8:44?

_____

_____

_____

According to 1 John 3:7-10, what is the difference between the children of God and the children of the devil?

_____

_____

_____

What is the warning found in 1 John 3:15?

_____

_____

_____

What is the ultimate destiny of the world in comparison to the destiny of the one who does the will of God?

_____

_____

_____

What hope for the believer can be found in 1 John 5:3-5,18-20?

_____

_____

_____

John 17 records the prayer of Jesus for Himself, His disciples and future believers. Read this chapter and consider this prayer of Jesus for you today. Respond to these words in your prayer journal today.

> *Lord, help me to recognize the world's influences on my emotions, mind, body and spirit. Teach me Your truth so I can recognize the devil's lies. Amen.*

CONFORMED OR TRANSFORMED?

*Father God, open my eyes that I might see where the world is
conforming me to its mold. May Your truth continue to transform
me as I study Your Word today. Amen.*

Have you ever considered the differences between "conform" and "transform"? The *Merriam-Webster Collegiate Dictionary* defines these words in this way:

Conform: to give the same shape, outline, or contour to: to bring into harmony or accord; to be similar or identical; to be obedient or compliant; synonym: "adapt"

Transform: to change in composition or structure; to change in character or condition; synonym: "convert" or "change"

Do you see the differences? What are the spiritual implications for each of these words based on our memory verse for this week?

Conform

_____

_____

_____

Transform

_____

_____

_____

What warnings concerning our fleshly desires are found in 1 Peter 1:14?

_____

_____

_____

In Ephesians 4:20-24, Paul instructs us in what it means to be transformed by Christ. What does Paul say controls the mind of the unbeliever (v. 22)? What does Paul say characterizes the life of a believer (vv. 23-24)?

_____

_____

_____

_____

According to 2 Corinthians 5:17, what occurred when we accepted Jesus Christ into our lives? In what ways have you experienced that process?

_____

_____

_____

_____

What does 2 Corinthians 3:18 say about the process of transformation? Who is doing the transforming?

_____

_____

_____

_____

Notice that Paul states we are *being transformed* into the likeness of Christ. This transformation takes time; in fact, for believers, becoming Christ-like is a lifelong process. As we stated in the introduction to this week's study, another word for this is "sanctification." To sanctify something or someone means to purify it, to make it holy, and to set it apart for a specific purpose. What is the promise found in 1 Thessalonians 5:23-24? Who is doing the sanctification?

_____

_____

_____

How have you seen the process of transformation happening in your life? In what ways are you a new creation?

_____

_____

_____

How have you seen the Lord at work in transforming you? Is there any area in your life in which you are resisting His transforming work?

_____

_____

_____

Thank You, Lord, that You are transforming me into the likeness of Christ. Give me the strength to resist the pull of my old self so that You can complete Your work of making me a new creation. Amen.

Day 3 — A NEW MIND

Lord, I want to have a renewed mind that is focused on You and Your truth. Please teach me how to achieve this as I continue to study Your Word. Amen.

Yesterday, we read in Ephesians 4:22-24 about where the battle between the old self and new self is being waged: primarily within our thoughts and our emotions. The world's intent is to make us look, act and/or think the same—to fit us into its mold. Just spend an evening watching television, leafing through a magazine or surfing the Internet to see how this world influences our thoughts and emotions.

How does Ephesians 4:17-19 describe the minds of unbelievers? (Note that the word "Gentiles" as used in this verse refers to unbelievers.)

_____

_____

_____

Read Romans 8:5-7. List how those with a sinful nature contrast with those who live in accordance with God's will.

Mind controlled by the sin nature	Mind controlled by the Spirit

What is the warning in Romans 8:9 and Galatians 6:7-8?

_____

_____

_____

According to Colossians 3:1-2, what are we to set our hearts and minds on? What are some practical ways we can do that when the sinful world continually tries to draw us away from God?

_____

_____

_____

Colossians 3:10 provides us with some instruction on how we can be renewed. The *New Living Translation* states it this way: "You have clothed yourselves with a brand-new nature that is continually being renewed as you learn more and more about Christ, who created this new nature in you." How can learning more and more about Christ renew your mind?

_____

_____

_____

What is the state of a mind focused on God as described in Isaiah 26:3 and John 14:27?

_____

_____

_____

What additional instruction about renewing your mind is found in Philippians 4:8?

_____

_____

_____

What is the result, according to verse 9?

_____

_____

_____

In what ways do you need the Lord to renew your mind?

_____

_____

_____

> *Lord, You have searched me and You know everything that goes on in my heart. If there is any way in which I am not focused on You, please point that out to me and lead me in Your way everlasting (see Psalm 139:1-2,23-24).*

Day 4

KNOWING GOD'S WILL

I admit, Lord, that I do not always understand Your will. Help me to learn more about You today. Amen.

In this week's Scripture memory verse, Paul states that we must be transformed by the renewing of our minds so that we will be able to "test and approve" what God's will is. But how can we "test and approve" God's will? In the *New Living Translation,* the phrase is translated, "Then you will know what God wants you to do." The *New American Standard Bible* translates it, "That you may prove what the will of God is." How do these translations shed light on the meaning of this phrase?

_____

_____

_____

What are your thoughts about God's will for your life? Fearful? Hopeful? Uncertain? Excited? Explain your choice.

_____

_____

_____

_____

According to 1 Thessalonians 4:3, what is God's will for you?

_____

_____

_____

Recall from the Day Two lesson what being "sanctified" means: to be purified, made holy and set apart for a specific purpose. How does that relate to knowing God's will?

_____

_____

_____

Read the following verses, and then note what each says about God's will.

Ephesians 5:15-18

_____

_____

_____

Philippians 2:12-13

_____

_____

_____

1 Thessalonians 5:18

_____

_____

_____

Read each of the following verses, and then note in the table below the way in which we are to discern the will of God.

Verse	How we are to discern God's will
Eph. 5:18	
Col. 1:9	
Jas. 1:5	

Through prayer, Bible study and the Holy Spirit living in us, we can better understand God and His will for our lives. Sometimes His will is hard to accept or to obey. What is the promise and blessing regarding God's will found in Hebrews 13:20-21?

_____

_____

_____

_____

I desire to do Your will, O my God. Your law is within my heart (see Psalm 40:8). Amen.

GOD'S GOOD, PLEASING AND PERFECT WILL

Day
5

*Help me, O God, to understand that Your will for me
is good, pleasing and perfect. Amen.*

Yesterday, we looked at how we can know God's will for our life. Today, we will take a closer look at God's will to determine how His purposes for us are always perfect and always have our best interests at heart. Begin by looking up Jeremiah 29:11-13. What is the promise found in this passage (v. 11)?

_____

_____

_____

_____

What is our part in this (vv. 12-13)?

_____

_____

_____

_____

In Hebrews 10:5-10, we read what Jesus said about doing God's will. What is the good news about doing God's will, according to verse 10?

_____

_____

_____

_____

What did Jesus say about God's will in John 6:38-40 that is also good news for believers?

_____

_____

_____

_____

How does 1 Corinthians 2:9 confirm God's loving will for us? From all of these verses, what do you understand about the immensity of God's love for you?

_____

_____

_____

_____

What did Jesus seek to do while here on earth, according to John 5:30?

_____

_____

_____

What is the promise found in 1 John 5:14?

_____

_____

_____

How does James 1:17 describe the gifts our heavenly Father gives us?

_____

_____

_____

Because of what you have learned these past two days, what conclusions can you make about God's will?

_____

_____

_____

_____

O Lord, fill me with the knowledge of Your will through all spiritual wisdom and understanding, in order that I might live a life pleasing to You and that I might bear fruit for You in every good work (see Colossians 1:9-10). Amen.

REFLECTION AND APPLICATION

Thank You, Lord, that You give me hope and that You are a trustworthy and loving God who has saved me from my sinful nature. Help me today to live in a way that honors You. Amen.

We have learned this week that the world has a different agenda for us than does God. This world wants to push us into a mold in which self is elevated above God and others. It encourages us to worship the prince of this world rather than the Creator of the whole universe. It leads us down a path paved with lies, destruction and death.

We have also learned that following God's plan for our lives will transform us into a new creation. God's path is paved with truth, good fruit and eternal life in heaven with our Lord and Savior. Jesus is the Good Shepherd who laid down His life for His sheep and leads us into righteousness and salvation.

In what ways have you seen God's transformation in each of the four aspects of your life? In what ways do you need His transforming power to work in these areas?

	How God has transformed me	Areas needing to be transformed
Spiritual		
Emotional		
Physical		
Mental		

It is only through God's transforming power that we can truly live balanced lives that bear eternal fruit. Do you remember the promise found in 1 Thessalonians 5:23-24? Pray that for yourself today.

> *O God of peace, sanctify me through and through. May my whole spirit,*
> *soul, mind and body be kept blameless at the coming of the Lord Jesus Christ.*
> *You have called me, and You are faithful to do what You have promised*
> *(see 1 Thessalonians 5:23-24). Amen!*

Day 7

REFLECTION AND APPLICATION

Thank You, heavenly Father, for what You have taught me from Your Word and through Your Holy Spirit this week. Show me how to take what I have learned and live it out in my life today and forever. Amen.

What better way is there to renew your mind than to study and memorize God's Word? It is the best way to test and approve what God's will is for your life. This week's memory verse gives specific instruction about how we can live holy lives in this sinful world. Romans 12:2 teaches us how to please God: We need to be transformed into new creatures with renewed minds so that we then can know His good, pleasing and perfect will.

As you do each day's study in *Seek God First*, there may be Scriptures that speak to you about a specific situation in your life, or a need you are experiencing or even a promise or blessing. If you haven't already done so, start writing down these special notes of love, encouragement and instruction from God on index cards, or on a special page in your journal or in a small notebook. Categorize them using labels such as "thanksgiving," "financial need," "fighting temptation" or any other categories you find helpful. In times of need, read through your Scripture collection. Begin to commit them to memory so you can recall them when you need them.

Having appropriate Scriptures available at your fingertips (or on the tip of your tongue) for use in any situation will provide you with a defense that is stronger than anything the enemy can throw in your path. The process of memorizing Scripture will also allow you to spend time with God even when you don't have your Bible available. Memorizing His Word and doing what it says are always pleasing to the Lord.

Father God, I know whom I believe in, and I am convinced that You are able to guard what I have entrusted to You (see 2 Timothy 1:12).

O God, thank You for granting me repentance and leading me to a knowledge of the truth! Thank You for bringing me to my senses so that I could escape from the trap of the devil, who had taken me captive to do his will (see 2 Timothy 2:25-26).

Father God, teach me, rebuke me and correct me through Your Word, which You inspired and have given to me, so that I may be fully equipped to do Your good work (see 2 Timothy 3:16-17).

Lord Jesus, help me to put on my new self, created to be like God in true righteousness and holiness (see Ephesians 4:24).

Dear heavenly Father, help me to no longer conform to the pattern of this world, but transform me by the renewing of my mind. Then will I be able to test and approve what Your will is for me: good, pleasing and perfect (see Romans 12:2).

Group Prayer Requests

4 first place health

Today's Date: _____

Name	Request

Results

_____

_____

_____

_____

_____

the dwelling place
of God

SCRIPTURE MEMORY VERSE
*Do you not know that your body is a temple of the Holy Spirit, who is
in you, whom you have received from God? You are not your own;
you were bought at a price. Therefore honor God with your body.*
1 CORINTHIANS 6:19-20

Our culture seems to worship the human body. We build up our bodies,
and we tear them down. We pamper them and then punish them with
torturous exercise. We sculpt them with plastic surgery and injections.
We show them off with scanty clothing. We tan, oil, peel, wax, pierce and
tattoo—all in the pursuit of the perfect body. The problem is that our
body worship honors the creation, not the Creator.

Perhaps our culture's focus on bodily perfection was what brought you
to First Place 4 Health. Are you striving for a perfect body, or are you working toward being a more healthy person who functions as God intended
with all four aspects of your being—physical, spiritual, emotional and men
tal—in balance? This week's study will walk us through the Scripture memory verse to discover what it means to honor God with our bodies.

YOUR BODY
Day 1

*O God, You created my body, soul, mind and emotions to bring honor
to You. Teach me through Your Word today. Amen.*

We will begin this lesson in some familiar territory: Psalm 139. This is a
psalm written by David celebrating how intimately our Creator knows

us. Read this psalm as a hymn of praise to your heavenly Father (aloud if possible). What do verses 13-14 specifically say about our bodies?

_____

_____

_____

Do you consider yourself "fearfully and wonderfully made"? You might look at your bodies and think, *Well, this body is not so wonderful. What happened, Lord?* But God has created you as a uniquely complex being with all the different components meant to work together in harmony. List some aspects about the workings of the human body that amaze you.

_____

_____

_____

_____

Unfortunately, this sinful fallen world takes its toll on these wonderfully crafted bodies that God has given us. In the world around us we see birth defects, genetic anomalies, illnesses, injuries and even the process of aging that bring about less than perfect bodies, and we might wonder why God would allow these things to happen. Remember that the evil one influences this world and that our lives on this earth are temporary. What is the promise about our earthly bodies found in Philippians 3:20-21?

_____

_____

_____

_____

What does Romans 12:1 say believers are to do with their bodies? How could this be a spiritual act of worship?

_____

_____

_____

Jesus was the ultimate sacrifice for our sin. What does Hebrews 7:27 say about Jesus' sacrifice?

_____

_____

_____

_____

What happened to the animals that were sacrificed in the Temple in Jerusalem (see Leviticus 17:11)? What does it mean to you to be a *living* sacrifice?

_____

_____

_____

_____

What new dimensions of the concept of being a living sacrifice does Paul add in Romans 6:11-14?

_____

_____

_____

How does knowing that your body is the temple of the Holy Spirit change your thinking about how you are to treat your own body?

_____

_____

_____

_____

Which of your behaviors are honoring God?

_____

_____

_____

_____

What attitudes about your body need to change in light of this week's Scripture memory verse and Romans 12:1?

_____

_____

_____

_____

Can you pray as Paul did in Philippians 1:20 that "now as always Christ will be exalted in my body"?

> *Marvelous Creator, I praise You because I have been fearfully and wonderfully made. Help me understand how I can be a living sacrifice for You and bring You honor and glory through the way I live out my faith in You. Amen.*

Day 2

GOD'S TEMPLE

Dear Lord, thank You for Your Holy Spirit's presence living in me. Teach me as I study today and continue my transformation into the person You have created me to be. Amen.

When the Early Christians were told that the believer was the temple of the Holy Spirit, they understood what that meant. Temples were a daily reality in their lives and an integral part of their history. What comes to your mind when you hear the word "temple"?

_____

_____

_____

_____

Examining the Temple in Jerusalem can give us a better understanding of what Paul meant when he used this word picture to describe our relationship with the indwelling Holy Spirit. As you read about the building of the Temple in 1 Kings 6:1-35, note the detailed descriptions. What do the details of these descriptions tell you about the importance of the Temple to our Lord God?

_____

_____

_____

There were three sections to the Temple building: (1) the outside porch, (2) the Holy Place and (3) the Most Holy Place. Hebrews 9:1-7 has a brief explanation of the different functions of the Holy Place (the outer room) and the Most Holy Place (the inner room). This passage primarily describes how the priests carried on their daily tasks in the outer room, but what does verse 7 say occurred once a year in the Most Holy Place?

_____

_____

_____

This sacrifice occurred annually on the Day of Atonement (Yom Kippur), when only the high priest could enter the Most Holy Place. What new dimension to this once-a-year sacrifice is added in Hebrews 9:11-14?

_____

_____

_____

Read Matthew 27:50-51. What happened to the veil that separated the Holy Place and the Most Holy Place in the Temple at the moment of Jesus' sacrificial death on the cross? What does that signify to you?

_____

_____

The Temple in Jerusalem was destroyed by the Romans in AD 70. Today, the Jews have no temple in which to perform the required sacrifices. The New Covenant brought about by Jesus' coming to earth, His death and

His resurrection have replaced the need for a manmade temple built of stones. First Peter 2:5 calls believers "living stones" that "are being built into a spiritual house." What do you think that spiritual house would be?

_____

_____

_____

Not only are believers the dwelling place of God's presence, but the Church is also referred to as God's temple. What information does 1 Corinthians 3:16-17 and Ephesians 2:21-22 give us about God's temple? (Note: The words translated as "you yourselves" in the *NIV* are in the plural, which signifies it is not referring to an individual but to a group of believers.)

_____

_____

_____

What new understanding have you come to concerning the significance of your body being the temple of God's Holy Spirit?

_____

_____

_____

Holy God, it is amazing that You would choose to live in me. Help me to live this day aware of the reality of Your presence dwelling in me. Today may You be glorified in my actions and words. Amen.

Day 3 — THE HOLY SPIRIT WITHIN

Thank You, Lord, for the gift of the Holy Spirit. I pray that He would teach me today. Amen.

As the third Person of the Trinity, the Holy Spirit is perhaps the most mysterious to believers. We can understand that we have a heavenly Father who sent His only Son in person to save us from our sins, but what about understanding the indwelling of the Holy Spirit in the believer? What did Jesus teach His disciples about the Holy Spirit in His Upper Room discourse as recorded in John 14:15-20?

_____

_____

_____

What additional information about the Holy Spirit, the Counselor, is given in John 16:7?

_____

_____

_____

Acts 2:1-11 describes what occurred when the disciples were given the gift of the Holy Spirit. How is the power of the Holy Spirit demonstrated in this scene? What is your reaction when you read this account?

_____

_____

_____

_____

Following this event, Peter preached the first evangelistic sermon in Acts 2:14-40. What was the result of Peter's sermon as recorded in verses 37 and 41? How was the power of the Holy Spirit displayed?

_____

_____

_____

According to verses 38-39, how does one receive the Holy Spirit?

_____

_____

_____

As you read the following verses, list what each says about the work of the Holy Spirit and note how it might be applied to your life.

Scripture	Work of the Holy Spirit	How it applies to my life
John 14:26		
John 15:26		
John 16:7-8		
Acts 9:31		
Rom. 8:26-27		
1 Cor. 2:9-13		
1 Cor. 12:3		

In Ephesians 4:30, Paul states, "Do not grieve the Holy Spirit of God, with whom you were sealed for the day of redemption." How might we grieve the Holy Spirit?

Lord, fill me with Your joy and peace as I trust in You so I might overflow with hope in the power of Your Holy Spirit. Help me to live this day in a way that does not grieve Your Holy Spirit who dwells within me. Amen.

Day 4 — PAID IN FULL

O Lord, help me to fully understand the cost that You paid for my salvation through Your death on the cross. Amen.

How is the worth of something determined? In our economic system, value is often determined by the price that the highest bidder will pay for an item. What does our memory verse say about the result of a price being paid for you?

_____

_____

_____

_____

What is your life worth? What is the price that was paid for it? To whom do we belong?

_____

_____

_____

What does Philippians 2:6-8 say about what Jesus gave up to come to earth to save us from our sins?

_____

_____

_____

According to Philippians 2:5, what should our reaction be to what the Lord gave up for us?

_____

_____

_____

To gain a better understanding of the value your heavenly Father has placed on your life, look up the following Scriptures and then note what each passage says about why you are valuable to God.

Scripture	Work of the Holy Spirit
Rom. 5:6-10	
Rom. 8:31-32	

Scripture	Work of the Holy Spirit
2 Cor. 8:9	
Gal. 1:3-4	
Gal. 2:20	
1 Tim. 2:5-6	
Titus 2:13-14	
Heb. 7:27	
1 John 2:1-2	

Considering the sacrificial price that was paid for you, are there any changes you need to make in your lifestyle? If so, what changes do you need to make?

_____

_____

_____

_____

What does Hebrews 13:15-16 say about the sacrifices that please God?

_____

_____

_____

In your prayer journal today, write a "sacrifice of praise" to the Lord about what He has done for you.

O Father God, it astounds me that You paid the supreme price: Your Son's death as the ransom for my sins. May my life be a sacrifice of praise today and every day. In the name of my Savior and Lord, amen.

HONOR GOD

*Show me, O God, how to apply Your Word to my life as I work
on my First Place 4 Health goals. Amen.*

In verse 20 of this week's Scripture memory verse, Paul writes, "Therefore honor God with your body." Perhaps you have heard it said that whenever we see the word "therefore" in Scripture, you need to ask yourself what it is "there for." In this passage, to what does the "therefore" refer? Why should we honor God with our bodies?

_____

_____

_____

In yesterday's lesson, we learned of the price that was paid for our bodies. How can we honor our Lord and Savior for the price He has paid?

_____

_____

_____

What does Romans 6:11-13 say about honoring God with our bodies?

_____

_____

_____

What is the warning found in Matthew 15:7-9?

_____

_____

_____

What does verse 8 say about what we should do to honor God?

_____

_____

_____

There are other ways in which we can honor God besides with our bodies. What does Proverbs 3:9 instruct us to do?

_____

_____

_____

According to 2 Corinthians 9:7, with what kind of attitude should we give?

_____

_____

_____

As you continue to read in 2 Corinthians 9:8-15, list the blessings that will result from your cheerful giving out of what the Lord has given you.

_____

_____

_____

How does cheerful giving relate to our giving honor to God?

_____

_____

_____

The last half of Proverbs 14:31 tells us of another action that honors God. How does this passage say we honor the Lord?

_____

_____

_____

In 1 Thessalonians 4:4, we are instructed to control our own bodies in a way that is holy and honorable. In what ways have you been successful in controlling your body?

_____

_____

_____

Where do you still struggle with self-control? In your prayer journal to-day, write about any struggles, and then write a prayer asking for God's power and strength to help you overcome your weaknesses. Pray believ-ing that you "can do all things through him who gives [you] strength" (Philippians 4:13).

> *"You are worthy, our Lord and God, to receive glory and honor and power, for You created all things, and by Your will they were created and have their being" (Revelation 4:11). Amen.*

REFLECTION AND APPLICATION

Day **6**

Almighty God, I pray for Your power and strength to build me into a temple worthy of Your presence. Amen.

Although the Lord wants you to have a healthy body, He is far more con-cerned about the sanctification process that comes from loving, knowing and obeying Him. As you go through the First Place 4 Health program, you will discover how to revitalize your physical body, strengthen your mind, renew your spirit and satisfy your emotional needs, but remember that any weight loss or healthy gain you might experience will come as a natural result of putting Christ first in your life. All the other blessings you will experience are just a bonus!

How have you seen the evidence of God's indwelling Spirit in your life?

_____

_____

In what ways have you been able to show honor to God through your First Place 4 Health participation?

_____

_____

What one action or change have you made as a result of this week's lesson?

_____

_____

_____

_____

What actions do you sense the Holy Spirit is leading you to take in living a more spiritually, physically, emotionally and mentally balanced life?

_____

_____

_____

_____

As you continue to seek God's will in your life, remember that the Holy Spirit is the Lord's empowering, encouraging and energizing force that is always at your disposal—living within you!

> *Thank You, Lord, for enabling me to live by Your Holy Spirit.*
> *Please help me to follow Your Spirit's leading in every part of my life*
> *(see Galatians 5:25). Amen.*

Day 7 REFLECTION AND APPLICATION

Dear God, please sanctify my body that through it I might bring honor to You. Thank You for the gifts of the Holy Spirit that make sanctification possible. Amen.

When Solomon built the Temple, he made it a beautiful place filled with gold and other precious materials. He wanted the whole world to see the beauty of the Temple and know that God's presence dwelt there. When God created humankind, He fashioned our bodies to be dwelling places for His Spirit. He wants the whole world to see you and know that His Holy Spirit lives inside.

Because God has chosen you to be a dwelling place for His Holy Spirit, you need to keep it filled with the good things that are pleasing and acceptable to Him. One of the best ways is to fill your heart and mind with His Word through Scripture memorization. As you are filled with His Word, you can't help but honor God in your whole being—body, soul, mind and emotions.

As you complete this week's Bible study, repeat the Scripture memory verse. Remember that each time you repeat the verse, God will plant this Scripture more firmly in your mind and heart. You will be enabled to live the sanctified life He has intended for you.

Lord Jesus, thank You for the promised Spirit of Truth who guides me into all truth so that I may understand You and Your Word (see John 16:13).

Thank You, Lord Jesus, that I have been made holy through the sacrifice of Your body, once for all (see Hebrews 10:10).

Dear heavenly Father, help me to remember that my body is a temple of Your Holy Spirit who I received from You and who now lives in me. I am not my own, because I was bought with the price—Jesus Christ's life was the ransom for my life. Therefore, I must honor You, O God, with my whole being (see 1 Corinthians 6:19-20). Amen.

Group Prayer Requests

4health
first place

Today's Date: _____

Name	Request

Results

_____

_____

_____

_____

_____

_____

commit to the Lord

SCRIPTURE MEMORY VERSE
*Commit to the LORD whatever you do,
and your plans will succeed.*
PROVERBS 16:3

Our society likes to measure success by the size of our bank accounts, or the model of car we drive, or the clothing we wear, or the gadgets we own, or the size of our homes. We plot our career tracks to bring about a successful lifestyle. Many parents are so concerned about the future success of their children that they plan every activity, event and even the schools they must attend. And did you know there is actually a magazine titled *SUCCESS*?

The toll from all this striving for success has been a lot of damage to our mental and physical health and to our relationships. We are a stressed-out society with untold billions of dollars going to help us deal with our overloaded bodies, minds and emotions. In fact, most of the serious health problems we face today are often related to the stress brought on by the pressure to succeed by the world's standards.

Not only is our society success oriented, but it also seems to be commitment-challenged. Have you ever planned a party and sent out invitations asking for RSVPs but received hardly any responses? It seems to be a sign of our times that people are even afraid to commit going to to a simple party! People seem afraid to commit to even the most worthwhile activity or relationship—unless it serves the purpose of furthering a personal agenda for their own success. After all, something better might come along.

God has a different definition of success than the world does. We have a holy God who requires a commitment to Him and His path for our lives to succeed. This week's lesson will explore what God's Word teaches us about success and commitment.

Day 1

DEFINING SUCCESS

O Lord, help me to understand success through Your eyes as I study Your Word. Amen.

Merriam-Webster's Collegiate Dictionary defines success as "a favorable or desired outcome; the attainment of wealth, favor, or eminence." How did you define success in your younger years?

_____

_____

_____

In what ways has your understanding of what determines success changed over the years? Why do you think it has changed?

_____

_____

_____

The Bible does not have one specific verse that states the definition of God's view of what success is, but we can get a sense of it from a few examples in Scripture. Read the parable of the rich fool in Luke 12:13-21. How does this parable relate to the world's definition of success?

_____

_____

_____

What is the warning found in verses 15 and 21?

_____

_____

_____

The verses following this parable might seem familiar to you. Scan Luke 12:22-34. What are the lessons found in these verses that relate to God's view of success?

_____

_____

_____

Do you know the story of Joseph in the Old Testament? Joseph was the favored son of Jacob. Because of his father's favor, Joseph's 10 older brothers hated him. One day they plotted to kill him, but instead they sold him into slavery. Read what happens in Genesis 39:1-6. How do verses 2 and 3 describe Joseph?

_____

_____

_____

Continue to read Genesis 39:7-23. Does Joseph seem successful now? He resisted temptation and was then falsely accused despite the fact that he was a good steward to his earthly master and obedient to the Lord. What is the final observation about Joseph made in verse 23?

_____

_____

_____

What does the story of Joseph tell you about God's definition of success?

_____

_____

_____

The word "prosper" is used in the Bible more often than the words "success" or "succeed." Read the following verses, and then match them to the observation about prosperity.

___ Deuteronomy 5:33	a.	Generosity brings prosperity.
___ Proverbs 11:25	b.	Concealed sin does not prosper.
___ Proverbs 19:8	c.	The one who seeks understanding prospers.
___ Proverbs 28:13	d.	Walk in the way of the Lord so that you may have prosperity and a long life.
___ Proverbs 21:21	e.	Pursuing righteousness and love brings life, prosperity and honor.

Joshua 1:8 states, "Do not let this Book of the Law depart from your mouth; meditate on it day and night, so that you may be careful to do everything written in it. Then you will be prosperous and successful." What does this verse say is the requirement for being prosperous and successful?

_____

_____

_____

Considering the verses you have studied, what would you say is the Lord's definition of "success"?

_____

_____

_____

How does this definition apply to your First Place 4 Health goals?

_____

_____

_____

Lord, help me to understand Your definition of success and how to attain it on Your terms. Amen.

THE BEST LAID PLANS

Day 2

*Father God, I commit this day to You and Your plans for me.
Keep me on Your path. Amen.*

Have you ever planned an event down to the last detail and had it either cancelled or just become a complete disaster? If so, you understand the saying, "The best laid plans of mice and men often go awry." One mistake that we as believers often make is that we make plans on our own and then ask the Lord to bless them. What do the following verses say about planning without consulting the Lord?

Scripture	Warning given
Ps. 33:10-11	
Prov. 19:21	
Prov. 27:1	
Isa. 30:1	
Jas. 4:13-15	

This does not mean that we are to forget about making plans and live moment by moment. We only need to look at the world God has created to recognize that He is a God of order and planning. He has an eternal plan in which we all have a part. Yes, He wants us to make plans, but in order to succeed at our plans we must be in tune with His will. Read 1 Chronicles 17:1-2. In this passage, King David had a dream to build the Temple in Jerusalem. Up until this time, the Ark of the Covenant did not have a permanent home. What do these verses tell us about David's motive for building the Temple? Does that seem like a good reason for his plan?

_____

_____

_____

What was the Lord's answer to David (vv. 5-14)?

_____

_____

_____

David responded to God's direction with praise and understanding (see 1 Chronicles 17:16-27). Then, in 1 Chronicles 22–29 we are given a description of all the preparations and plans that David provided so that Solomon could begin building the Temple after David's death. According to 1 Chronicles 22:6-9, what was David's explanation to Solomon for why the Lord would not allow him to realize this dream?

_____

_____

_____

_____

David had what seemed like a good idea to him—to build a permanent Temple to glorify God—and yet God stopped him. So instead, David set about preparing the materials and the people to build a magnificent structure that he would never see. What do you suppose would have happened if David had ignored the Lord and continued on with his desire to build the Temple himself?

_____

_____

_____

_____

Did you notice that even Nathan, God's prophet and David's spiritual advisor, initially told David to go ahead with his plans (see 1 Chronicles 17:2), but then God spoke to Nathan in a dream telling him to stop David (see v. 4)? It is good to consult fellow believers for advice on our plans, but remember that ultimately we must commit our plans to the Lord for them to succeed. Of course, there will be times when we won't understand the reason that God does not approve of what seems like a worthy plan. How can Isaiah 55:8-9 help us to understand why this happens?

_____

_____

_____

_____

Have you ever had an experience in which the Lord thwarted your plans and then, when you looked back, you realized that there was a really good reason that those plans were not carried out? If so, describe what happened. What did you learn from the experience?

_____

_____

_____

_____

Although we don't always want to admit it, our heavenly Father really does know best!

> *Lord, Your Word tells me that You know the plans You have for me,*
> *plans to prosper me and not to harm me, plans to give me hope and a*
> *future (see Jeremiah 29:11). I cling to those words of promise*
> *now as I ask for Your direction for my life. Amen.*

COMMIT TO THE LORD   Day 3

Lord, I commit this day to You and to the study of Your Word. I need
Your wisdom and understanding as I read. Amen.

In Mark 8:34-35, Jesus states, "If anyone would come after me, he must deny himself and take up his cross and follow me. For whoever wants to save his life will lose it, but whoever loses his life for me and for the gospel will save it." It is easy to say that we believe in the Lord Jesus Christ and even that we want Him to live in us. What does this passage say about true commitment to the Lord? What warnings are given in verses 36-38?

_____

_____

_____

This command was so important that it was repeated three more times in the Gospels (see Matthew 10:38; 16:24; Luke 9:23). What does this command mean to you and your commitment?

_____

_____

_____

Sometimes there are strongholds that hinder our complete commitment to the Lord. In 1 Samuel 7:1-3, we read about the return of the Ark of the Covenant to Israel after a 20-year absence. What was Samuel's challenge to the Israelites in verse 3? What was the people's response in verse 4?

_____

_____

_____

What might the "foreign gods and the Ashtoreths" be compared to in our lives today?

_____

_____

_____

What is it that hinders your commitment to follow God wholeheart-edly? How will you commit to putting away these things from your life?

_____

_____

_____

_____

During this study, we have often discussed how each of us has both major and minor choices to make every day. Today, you have a choice to make regarding commitment to God's plan for your life—and this choice will have a consequence. In the next two days' lessons, we will look at some of the consequences of choosing to rebel or to willingly follow God's will.

Dear Lord, it is often hard for me to relinquish control, but I know that You have a better plan for me. Help me to seek Your plan for today. Amen.

A REBELLIOUS ATTITUDE

Day 4

O Lord, expose any rebellious attitudes that I might have toward following Your commands. Thank You, Lord. Amen.

In Numbers 13, we read the story of how God appointed 12 men from the tribes of Israel to go and investigate the land that He had promised to deliver into their hands. When 10 of the spies came back and reported that the people who lived in the land were powerful and that the Israelites couldn't win a battle against them, the Lord sent them to wander in the wilderness for 40 years. During their years of wandering, the Israelites repeatedly rebelled against the Lord.

Psalm 78 gives a summary of the cycles of rebellion of the people as they wandered in the desert. What were some of the things God did for the Israelites listed in verses 12-16?

_____

_____

_____

What rebellious acts of the people are listed in verses 17-20?

_____

_____

_____

What were some of the actions that God took against the people when they were rebellious (see vv. 21,31,33)?

_____

_____

_____

What did He do when they repented (see vv. 38-39)?

_____

_____

_____

What is the indictment against rebellion found in 1 Samuel 15:22-23?

_____

_____

_____

To further understand this indictment, what does Deuteronomy 18:9-12 say about those who practice divination?

_____

_____

_____

Today, think about your motives for participating in First Place 4 Health. Trying to lose weight or exchanging healthy habits for unhealthy ones are good goals to have, but whenever we strike out on our own to change our behaviors, we will fail without God's help. In your prayer journal, write a prayer of confession for any acts of rebellion you may have committed in your life, and make a commitment to follow God's will in all things for your life.

> *O Father God, show me where I need to change my attitude about obeying You. Thank You for Your grace and mercy in dealing with any rebellious actions that I have committed. Amen.*

A WILLING ATTITUDE

Gracious Lord, I ask today that You give me a willing spirit to do what You have commanded me to do. Amen.

God only wants the best for us, but sometimes we may feel rebellious because we want to be the one in control. In these instances, we need to remember that God's control is not meant to chain us down to difficult rules but to set us free to enjoy the life He has planned for us. Furthermore, when we are rebellious to God's will, He will discipline us. Our attitude toward God's discipline will make a big difference in how successful we will be at changing our lifestyle and being obedient to God.

According to Hebrews 12:5-6, how should you respond when God disciplines you?

_____

_____

_____

_____

What does God's discipline accomplish in your life according to Hebrews 12:10-11?

_____

_____

_____

_____

Look up the following passages of Scripture and note what are the rewards of a willing attitude that delights in the Lord:

Psalm 1:1-3

_____

_____

_____

Psalm 37:3-6

_____

_____

_____

Psalm 143:10

_____

_____

_____

Proverbs 3:5-6

_____

_____

_____

Have you experienced delight in following God? If so, give an example.

_____

_____

_____

_____

Do you struggle with following the Lord wholeheartedly? If so, what promise does each of the following verses give you?

Psalm 28:7

_____

_____

_____

Jeremiah 33:3

_____

_____

_____

Philippians 4:13

_____

_____

_____

Perhaps willing commitment to the Lord is a new experience for you. If so, pray today's closing prayer, which David wrote in Psalm 51 after he was disciplined by the Lord for his sin with Bathsheba.

> *Create in me a pure heart, O God, and renew a steadfast spirit within me. Restore to me the joy of Your salvation and grant me a willing spirit to sustain me (see Psalm 51:10,12). Amen.*

REFLECTION AND APPLICATION

Day 6

Precious Lord, I want a willing spirit that delights in the time I spend with You in reading Your Word and in conversation. Refresh me today as I consider what I have learned this week. Amen.

Do you realize that when you began this study and your participation in First Place 4 Health, you made a commitment to follow God's leading and to put Christ first in your life? Today, take a few moments to really consider that commitment you made to God as you have worked through this study. In the following scale, place an X on the line to indicate the degree of success you have achieved toward each goal or commitment (1 being the lowest degree of success and 5 being the highest).

Prayer	1 _____	5
Bible study	1 _____	5
Scripture memory	1 _____	5
Group accountability	1 _____	5
Nutrition plan	1 _____	5
Exercise	1 _____	5
Daily Tracker	1 _____	5

Do not be discouraged if you feel that you haven't quite met your goals in the way that you would have liked. You cannot change a pattern of poor habits and unhealthy choices overnight! Where do you sense that God is leading you to put more of an emphasis into the changes you need to make?

_____

_____

_____

_____

_____

What will you plan (with the Lord's guidance) to do now to start making that change?

_____

_____

_____

_____

What promises in Matthew 11:28-30 can you apply to following God's plan for your life?

_____

_____

_____

_____

We can always put our trust in the Lord's plan. He only wants the best for us. He has given us guidelines for following His way of life. We just need to commit our plans to Him and watch them succeed.

O gracious Lord, thank You that when I take Your yoke upon me, I will know Your gentleness and humility and it will bring rest to my soul. Thank You that Your yoke is easy and Your burden is light. Don't let me pick up any burden that is not mine (see Matthew 11:28-30). Amen.

REFLECTION AND APPLICATION

*Lord, I commit this lesson to reflecting on what You have taught me
this week and to applying what I've learned to my life. Amen.*

This week, we have discussed committing our plans to God. The keys to properly following God's will are studying God's Word each day, spending time in prayer, and reading and memorizing Scripture. It is only through focusing our lives first on the *spiritual* actions that we will succeed in all the other aspects of our lives.

If you have fallen behind in any of those areas, don't give up! Begin anew by making the commitment to spend regular, consistent time with the Lord. Even if you can only spend 5 to 10 minutes in prayer or Bible Study at first, start there. Even on the busiest days, a few moments with the Lord will bring other things in your life into line.

During your times of prayer, the verses from the Bible studies will help you seek God's guidance. Remember that they represent the sword of the Spirit and that they are more powerful against Satan than any other weapon you might have at your disposal.

Throughout *Seek God First*, Day 7 of each week's Bible study has ended with a prayer written from the memory verse for that week. Review those prayers and use them in your own prayer time to strengthen your desire to follow God's plan for your life. You should be well on your way to overcoming any strongholds that threaten to keep you from following God's will for your life, so don't be discouraged if you happen to slip, for God is your refuge and fortress. Go to Him with your disappointments, anger, resentment, guilt, depression or whatever might threaten your walk with Him. He will be with you and will help you overcome any obstacles.

My faithful Father, whether I turn to the right or to the left, cause my ears to hear a voice behind me saying, "This is the way; walk in it" (see Isaiah 30:21).

Lord, I commit to You everything that I do because I know You will help me to succeed (see Proverbs 16:3).

Group Prayer Requests

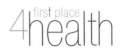

Today's Date: _____

Name	Request

Results

_____

_____

_____

_____

_____

_____

God is love!

SCRIPTURE MEMORY VERSE

A new command I give you: Love one another. As I have loved you, so you must love one another. By this all men will know that you are my disciples, if you love one another.

JOHN 13:34-35

What thoughts or images come to mind when you hear the word "love"? Watch a couple of hours of television or a popular movie and you will see that the most common plot seems to be the pursuit of romantic love or the lack thereof. Even an exciting adventure story often has a romantic undercurrent to it.

In our culture, we use love to describe a feeling about the most trivial of matters. We say things like, "I *love* mocha almond fudge" or "I *love* that dress on you." We have even adopted the ♥ symbol to substitute for the word so we don't have to write the whole word. It seems that everyone ♥s almost anything from their pets to their hobbies!

Loving and being loved in return is a basic human need. When love is denied or lost, it can have an emotionally devastating effect on our lives. In fact, children placed in orphanages where they do not get regular loving attention have been known to waste away and even to die. Without love, life is hardly worth living. Fortunately, we have a Savior who loves us so much that He died for us so that we might live with Him forever!

In this week's study, we will consider Jesus' command that we love one another and examine how that command is related to the love He has demonstrated for us.

DEFINING LOVE

*O heavenly Father, You are the source of all love. Show me how
to express love to You. Amen.*

As we mentioned in the introduction to this week's study, the English
word "love" is used to describe all different kinds of emotions or passions. We use it to express our affection toward other people. We use it
to express romantic love or sexual passion. We also use it to designate
our emotional ties to family members and friends. "Love" expresses our
feelings for a pet, a cause, a pastime, a celebrity, a sports team or even
possessions. It's even used as a scoring term in tennis!

However, the Hebrew and Greek languages (the two languages in
which the majority of the Bible was written) use several different words
to describe the various different aspects of love. In the Hebrew language,
there are two words that are primarily translated as the word "love" in
English versions of the Bible. The first word is *hesed*, which usually refers
to unfailing or loyal love, devotion or kindness. This word is primarily
used to indicate the love that God has for us.[1] The second word, *'ahab*,
refers to the kind of love that humans are capable of, including our re-
ciprocal love for or toward God. It is also used to indicate love of friends
and family as well as romantic love.[2]

Read Psalm 119:41,47,48,64 and 76. Consider the above definitions, and
then determine which of these words are being used in each instance.

v. 41	☐ hesed	☐ 'ahab
v. 47	☐ hesed	☐ 'ahab
v. 48	☐ hesed	☐ 'ahab
v. 64	☐ hesed	☐ 'ahab
v. 76	☐ hesed	☐ 'ahab

In Greek, the language of the New Testament, there are three main forms
of the word that are usually translated into English as the word "love,"
two of which are used in the Bible. The first word is *agape* (noun form)

and *agapeo* (verb form), which refers to the active love God has for His Son and His people and the active love His people are to have for Him, each other and even enemies. It denotes sacrificial love.[3] The second word, *phileo,* refers to affection and regard of a high order.[4] It is the root word in *philadelphia,* which means brotherly love and kindness.[5] (The third word for "love" not used in the Bible is *eros,* which refers to sexual or romantic love.)

Look at this week's memory verses. What form of the Greek word for "love" do you suppose is used in this passage? Based on the above definitions, why do you think this is the case?

_____

_____

_____

If you chose *agapeo,* you are correct. In fact nearly all the words translated as "love" in the New Testament are a form of *agape* or *agapeo.* What does that tell you about the focus of love in the New Testament?

_____

_____

_____

Agape love is defined by God's love for us. What is the ultimate evidence of God's love for us, according to Romans 5:8?

_____

_____

_____

First Corinthians 13 (known as the "love chapter") gives us some practical examples of the meaning of *agape* love. Although this chapter is often read at weddings to remind the bride and groom about how to love one another, it is not just intended for newlyweds—it is intended for all of us! Read verses 4-8 from this chapter, and then note in the following table what Paul says love is and what it is not.

Verse	What love is	What love is not
v. 4		
v. 5		
v, 6		
v. 7		
v. 8		

In 1 Corinthians 13:1-3, Paul makes several comparisons to good things that go bad without love. As you read these verses, answer the following questions, giving specific examples if possible:

How can speaking in holy words sound like a clanging gong without love (v. 1)?

_____

_____

_____

How can the gifts of prophecy, preaching and imparting knowledge and faith accomplish nothing if performed without love (v. 2)?

_____

_____

_____

How can giving to the poor or even dying for a good cause be considered nothing when done without love (v. 3)?

_____

_____

_____

God has certainly redefined the meaning of love in our vocabulary. In fact, 1 John 4:16 declares that "God *is* love." Today, think about how you are enacting this type of love in your relationships with others.

Lord God, as the psalmists wrote, "Your love endures forever" (see Psalm 136). I thank You that Your love never fails and that You have given us Jesus to demonstrate that love. Help me to pass Your love on to others today. Amen.

A NEW COMMAND

Day 2

O Lord, You have commanded me to love others. Help me to understand what that means and to act on that understanding. Amen.

This week's memory verse states that Jesus was giving His disciples a new command to "love one another." Have you ever wondered why He called this a *new* command? After all, this law was first stated to the Israelites in Leviticus 19:18. What was the specific instruction in that verse?

_____

_____

_____

_____

There is one other time this command appears—in Leviticus 19:34. Who is the specific "neighbor" being mentioned here? What was the Lord's reason that these particular people should be shown love?

_____

_____

_____

There are only a few other times (for instance, in Deuteronomy 10:19) that the Lord commanded the Israelites to love the foreigners among them, and it was always to be done in connection with being *kind* and *helpful* to them. In addition, there are several places in the Old Testament where the Israelites were instructed to show *kindness* and *care* for those in need (to widows and orphans in particular). There is another aspect in which this command to love one another would have been new to the disciples: In the Leviticus and Deuteronomy passages, the Hebrew word translated as "love" is *'ahab*. Based on yesterday's lesson, what kind of love does that word denote?

Throughout the Old Testament, whenever God commands the people to love Him or each other, the word *'ahab* is used. However, whenever God speaks of His love for His people, the word *hesed* is used. Do you see the interesting distinction here? What does this seem to signify?

The Greek word for love that is used in our memory verse is *agapeo*. Once again, what does this form of the word "love" mean?

From this, we can determine that when Jesus commanded His disciples to love one another as He loved them, He was telling them to love one another with a godly love that can only come through His Holy Spirit who dwells within them. This was revolutionary—a new level of love! One last distinction that makes this command unique is that Jesus was commanding them to love *each* other, as He loved them. This was not a command for them to love unbelievers (although this is commanded elsewhere), but for them to love *fellow believers*. Jesus restated this command in John 15:12,17. That's three times in just two chapters! What does the repetition of the command to "love one another" mean to you?

How many times is the command to love one another made in John 13:34-35? Once again, what is the significance of that repetition?

_____

_____

_____

Our love for fellow believers is a high priority to Jesus. What will be the hoped-for result of this love between believers, according to verse 35? How have you experienced this in your own life?

_____

_____

_____

What added dimensions about loving fellow believers are found in the following verses?

Romans 12:9-10,13

_____

_____

_____

Galatians 6:9-10

_____

_____

_____

As you conclude today's study, think of the ways in which you and your group members show the love of Christ to each other. What are some ways group members have shown God's love to you?

_____

_____

_____

In what ways have you shown love to group members?

_____

_____

_____

> *Thank You, Jesus, that You have shown Your love for me. Help me to extend that love to others, especially those in my First Place 4 Health group. Amen.*

Day 3

AS JESUS HAS LOVED US

Thank You, Jesus, that You have loved me so much that You gave Your life for me. Show me how to love others the way that You do. Amen.

In yesterday's lesson, we read in John 15:12 that Jesus told His disciples a second time to love one another. What does verse 13 tell us about the ultimate demonstration of this love for one another?

_____

_____

_____

According to 1 John 3:16, what action shows us the meaning of *agape* love?

_____

_____

_____

What further instruction is given in verses 17-18 on how to show love to our fellow believers?

_____

_____

_____

The book of 1 John uses the various forms of *agape* and *agapeo* 43 times (in the fourth chapter alone, these words are used 32 times). Read 1 John

4:7-10. What do these verses say about how God demonstrated His love for us?

_____

_____

_____

What promises are found in verses 15-17?

_____

_____

_____

Can you fathom the kind of love God has for you? How can it be possible to love others the way that God loves us, according to Romans 5:5?

_____

_____

_____

Loving others unconditionally is not an easy task, but remember that God loves everyone—believer and nonbeliever alike. We need to see others through the compassionate eyes of Jesus and learn to love as He first loved us. He has sent His Holy Spirit to dwell in us and to give us the strength and ability to love even the most unlovable.

Lord, I praise You for sending Your Son into the world that I might live through Him. Help me to live this day with that knowledge deeply engrained in my soul. May Your Holy Spirit empower me to show Your love to others. Amen.

LOVING OTHERS — Day 4

Dear Lord, help me to see the needs of others through Your eyes. Help me to love others with the same love You have poured into me by Your Holy Spirit. Amen.

In Mark 12:28-34, we read how one of the teachers of the law approached Jesus as He was speaking and asked Him a pointed question about exactly what was the most important commandment to God. What was Jesus' answer (vv. 30-31)?

_____

_____

_____

In Mark 12:30-31, we encounter a familiar verse, one that is at the core of First Place 4 Health. Beside loving God with all our heart, soul, mind and strength, who else are we to love? What can we conclude from the order of the list of those whom we are to love?

_____

_____

_____

God is first on our list of those to whom we are to show love, followed by loving our neighbors. What does 1 John 4:21 say about loving both God and others?

_____

_____

_____

According to Luke 10:25-37, how can we be a good neighbor?

_____

_____

_____

What are some practical ways we can show love to others, according to Colossians 3:12-14?

_____

_____

_____

_____

Who else are we to love, according to Matthew 5:43-47?

_____

_____

_____

_____

Nowhere in the Old Testament is there an instruction to hate our enemies, but it had become a part of the Jewish tradition, and thus it was considered acceptable to do so. What additional instructions about how to treat your enemies are found in the following verses?

Luke 6:27-36

_____

_____

_____

Romans 12:17-21

_____

_____

_____

Is there someone in your life who rubs you the wrong way or stresses you out by his or her behavior? If so, begin to pray for your relationship with that person and ask God to allow you to shine the light of His love into it. At first this may seem impossible to do, but remember that you are not relying on your own strength but on the strength and power of the Holy Spirit within you. Write out a prayer asking God to help you forgive this person for the hurts of the past, and ask Him to give you the supernatural *agape* love you will need in order to love this person sincerely. It will not happen overnight, but with God's grace and persistence, you can do it!

Dear Lord Jesus, You have loved me with a love I cannot fathom. Let Your love shine through me to those who need Your loving grace and mercy. Amen.

THAT OTHERS MAY KNOW

Father God, it is only through Your grace and power that I can love others unconditionally. You have told me that You will provide what I ask for, so I am asking for Your grace and power to love. Amen.

According to John 3:16, how did God demonstrate His love for us?

_____

_____

_____

_____

What is the extent of God's love, as recorded in John 3:17? Who is included within the circle of His love?

_____

_____

_____

_____

In Matthew 5:14-16, Jesus described how believers are His light for this world. How can our showing His love to others be a light to the world? What will be the result when we shine God's love on others?

_____

_____

_____

_____

Before Christ left this earth and ascended into heaven, He gave a charge to His disciples. Read His words in Matthew 28:19-20. How is obeying this commandment related to loving our neighbors—and even our enemies?

_____

_____

_____

_____

How did you come to know and trust Jesus Christ as Your Savior? Who shared the gospel message with you? How did you see God's light through that person (or those persons)?

_____

_____

_____

How might your participation in First Place 4 Health shine a beacon of God's love to the world around you?

_____

_____

_____

Sharing God's gospel message with others is the ultimate expression of His *agape* love. Who in the circle of people that you know need to know about the love of Christ? Are you praying for them to come to know Him? In what ways can you show them God's love? If you haven't already done so, write a list of people in your prayer journal for whom you are praying to receive Jesus as their Lord and Savior. Pray for them daily and ask the Lord to give you specific ways that you can share His love with them.

> *O Lord, may the light of Your love in me so shine before others that they would see the good works I do in Your name and glorify You. I pray that others might come to know You through the light of Your love in me. Amen.*

REFLECTION AND APPLICATION

Day
6

> *Dear Lord, I pray that You would strengthen me today through the power of Your Spirit. Help me to fully grasp the reality of Your love. Amen.*

We can have head knowledge about God's love and yet fail to grasp the reality of that love. A total understanding of God's love for us and the whole world is beyond our human comprehension, yet we must continually try to comprehend this type of love in order for our faith to grow.

In Ephesians 3:15-21, Paul gives us a glimpse of the scope of God's love. Meditate on these verses, and then answer the following questions.

Who can be included in the expanse of God's love (v. 15)?

_____

_____

_____

_____

How long will God keep loving the world? How long will He keep loving you (v. 21)?

_____

_____

_____

How does the cross remind you of the heights God's love will reach?

_____

_____

_____

_____

God, the Creator of the universe, totally loves us as we are. Of course, this doesn't mean that He loves everything we do, but He does love us as completely. In fact, He loves us too much to let us stay in the place that we are—He wants us to be continually learning about Him and growing in our faith. That fact should revolutionize our lives as we continue to put Him in first place in all things. Today, write a prayer of praise in your journal for His infinite love and renew your commitment to following the Lord wholeheartedly.

> *Lord, grant me the power to grasp how wide and long and high and deep is the love of Christ. Help me to know Your love that surpasses knowledge so I may be filled to the measure of all the fullness of God (see Ephesians 3:18-19).*

REFLECTION AND APPLICATION

Thank You, Jesus, for Your love and the sacrifice that You made for me on the cross. May I grasp the depth of Your love today and pass it on to others. Amen.

You have reached the last day of Bible study for this session. Throughout this study, the emphasis has been on giving Christ first place in your heart, mind, soul and body. You have learned how to pray, how to joyfully obey, how to please God, how to experience contentment, how to resist temptation and how to value your body and take care of it. Each week, the memory verse has pointed you toward giving Christ first place in your life. As you conclude this study, reflect on what you have learned about yourself and about God the Father, God the Son *and* God the Holy Spirit.

The goals of First Place 4 Health are not just for you to pursue while you are in a Bible study. Rather, continually strive to make them a part of your daily life whether you're enrolled in a session or not. A life filled with Bible study, Scripture memorization, prayer, healthy eating, exercise and encouragement to others will keep you close to Him and feeling better about yourself. In addition, a life centered on the Lord will be a beacon of His love that shines on others so that they will want to know Him as well.

Holy Lord, I am convinced that neither death nor life, neither angels nor demons, neither the present nor the future, nor any powers, neither height, nor depth, nor anything else in all creation, will be able to separate me from the love of God that comes through Christ Jesus my Lord (see Romans 8:38-39). Help me to love others as You have loved me. Let all know that I am Your disciple through my love for others (see John 13:34-35).

Notes

1. Edward W. Goodrick and John R. Kohlenberger III, *Strong's NIV Exhaustive Concordance* (Grand Rapids, MI: Zondervan, 1999), Hebrew #2876.
2. Ibid., Hebrew #170 and 173.
3. Ibid., Greek #26 and #27.
4. Ibid., Greek #5797.
5. Ibid., Greek #5789.

Group Prayer Requests

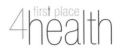

Today's Date: _____

Name	Request

Results

_____
_____
_____
_____
_____
_____

time to
celebrate!

To help shape your brief victory celebration testimony, work through the following questions in your prayer journal:

Day One: List some of the benefits you have gained by allowing the Lord to transform your life through this 12-week First Place 4 Health session. Be sure to list benefits you have received in the physical, mental, emotional and spiritual realms of your being.

Day Two: In what ways have you most significantly changed *mentally*? Have you seen a shift in the ways you think about yourself, food, your relationships or God? How has Scripture memory been a part of these shifts?

Day Three: In what ways have you most significantly changed *emotionally*? Have you begun to identify how your feelings influence your relationship to food and exercise? What are you doing to stay aware of your emotions, both positive and negative?

Day Four: In what ways have you most significantly changed *spiritually*? How has your relationship with God deepened? How has drawing closer to Him made a difference in the other three areas of your life?

Day Five: In what ways have you most significantly changed *physically*? Have you met or exceeded your weight/measurement goals? How has your health improved the past 12 weeks?

Day Six: Was there one person in your First Place 4 Health group who was particularly encouraging to you? How did their kindness make a difference in your First Place 4 Health journey?

Day Seven: Summarize the previous six questions into a one-page testimony, or "faith story," to share at your group's victory celebration.

May our gracious Lord bless and keep you as you continue to keep Him first in all things!

Seek God First
leader discussion guide

For in-depth information, guidance and helpful tips about leading a successful First Place 4 Health group, spend time studying the *First Place 4 Health Leader's Guide*. In it, you will find valuable answers to most of your questions as well as personal insights from many First Place 4 Health group leaders.

For the group meetings in this session, be sure to read and consider each week's discussion topics several days before the meeting—some questions and activities require supplies and/or planning to complete. Also, if you are leading a large group, plan to break into smaller groups for discussion and then come together as a large group to share your answers and responses. Make sure to appoint a capable leader for each small group so that discussions stay focused and on track (and be sure each group records their answers!).

week one: welcome to *Seek God First*

During this first week, welcome the members to your group, provide a brief overview of the First Place 4 Health program, explain what is expected of the participants at each of the weekly meetings, and collect the Member Surveys. (See the *First Place 4 Health Leader's Guide* for a detailed outline of how to conduct the first week's meeting.)

week two: first things first

As you and the group begin to work through the *Seek God First* Bible study, be mindful that there may be those in your group who have not done a focused Bible study before. Be sure to take some time at the beginning of this week's lesson to explain the importance of daily Bible study as an integral part of First Place 4 Health.

Discuss what the members discovered when they looked at the entries in their calendar or checkbook. What did this tell them about the areas they have been giving first place in their lives? What are some of the concerns that tend to divert their attention from Jesus' priorities in their lives?

Discuss some of the items the members listed that cause them to worry. Talk about the positive action they can take according to Philippians 4:6-7 when they find themselves worrying about something.

Ask someone to read Romans 14:17. Discuss the two items this passage lists that are not priorities to God and the three items that are. Talk about how the non-priorities relate to our physical lives while the priorities relate to our spiritual lives.

Talk about Jesus, the great high priest, the One who intercedes for us. Discuss how Jesus was tempted in every way just as we are and what that means for us. Ask your group what weaknesses they need to bring to the great high priest today, and then lead a time of prayer to present these needs before the throne of grace.

Discuss some of the attributes the members listed from the Day 5 study that defines one who places the Lord first in his or her life. Talk about what the participants discovered when they did the exercise in which they examined the degree to which they put Christ first in various aspects of their lives.

Ask the members what they learned this week about putting Christ in first place in each of the four core areas of their lives. Discuss what areas of strength and what areas of weakness they discovered. Conclude in prayer, asking God to break any strongholds in the members' lives.

week three: let's pray

Begin the discussion with group prayer, asking for a couple of volunteers to lead in prayer. Ask group members to share their responses to the description of the holiness of God. Discuss why we can now approach the throne of almighty God with confidence. Discuss what the group members learned from Jesus' example of praying. Then invite volunteers to share some of their ideas for when they pray and where they pray.

On a flipchart or whiteboard, write the acrostic letters A-S-K down the left side. Then ask the group what each letter stands for according to Matthew 7:7-9 (**A**sk, **S**eek, **K**nock). Discuss how each word applies to prayer and write their suggestions next to each word.

Discuss what conditions might block our prayers and relate this to the conditions that have positive results for our prayer. Encourage one or two volunteers to tell about lessons they have learned about prayers being answered.

On Day 4 there was a matching activity to complete. Have group members share their matches. Discuss the importance of learning to forgive to promote good spiritual, mental, emotional and even physical health. Ask group members to share some of their creative ways to pray from the activity on Day 6. As they share, write the ideas on the flipchart or whiteboard. Invite a few volunteers to share their experiences as they tried their creative suggestions.

Complete the discussion by inviting volunteers to share if they have had an experience where knowing Scripture has helped them to pray. Ask group members to recite the five aspects of prayer that were discussed in this week's lesson (*adoration, surrender, supplication, confession, protection*), writing the words on the flipchart or whiteboard. Close the discussion time with prayer by mentioning each word and allowing the members to respond by using that aspect in short phrases or single words of prayer.

week four: blessed obedience

As you begin this lesson, discuss the question: "Why is obedience so difficult for us?" Write the group's comments on a flipchart or whiteboard. If no one else suggests it, point out that we want to control our own lives. Lead into a discussion of why obedience is good for us.

Discuss the example of Jesus' obedient attitude. Some might say it was easy for Jesus to be obedient since He was God, but help them realize that He was human while here on earth and how He accepted the limitations. Refer to the Scriptures about His agony in the Garden of Gethsemane as He wrestled with obedience that would lead to His death as evidence that obedience was not easy for Him.

Point out that being obedient is a daily choice—a choice that we can make reluctantly or willingly. Invite volunteers to share some of the thoughts that might keep them from obeying the Lord. Discuss how we might overcome those negative thoughts.

On the flipchart or whiteboard, write "The Costs" across the top on the left side. Draw a line down the length of the paper or board. On the right side of the line across the top write "The Rewards." Ask group members to share what are the costs of disobedience and write them under that heading. After several have shared, do the same for the rewards of obedience. Invite volunteers to share about which reward is most appealing.

Relate obeying God to their full participation in the First Place 4 Health program. Discuss what the benefits of each aspect of the program are: Scripture reading, prayer, Bible study, Scripture memory, group accountability, nutrition plan, exercise, and daily tracker. Encourage group members to persevere, reminding them of these benefits.

Discuss why we should obey those in authority over us and how that is honoring to God. If appropriate, stop right now and pray for those who struggle with difficult authorities in their lives. Conclude by discussing what the members wrote on their Day 6 summaries of what they learned about obedience in all aspects of their lives.

week five: there's no excuse

Begin this lesson by reading Genesis 3:1-6. Discuss the lies that Satan used to deceive Eve and how that applies to the temptations we face today. Discuss why God gave Adam and Eve the opportunity to choose whether or not to obey His command.

Invite a volunteer to read Genesis 3:7-11; then discuss why Adam and Eve felt the need to hide from God after their disobedience, why God asked where they were, and why they had disobeyed Him. If the discussion does not bring it about, point out that God gives us free will so that we are not merely robots; He wants us to come to Him by choice, not by force.

Turn the discussion to the excuses that were made, first Adam's and then Eve's. Point out that Adam was subtly blaming God for giving Eve to him and that he pushed the blame on to Eve who then shifted the blame to the serpent. Ask group members to share some unusual excuses they have heard for someone's indiscretions. (Note: Instruct them not to use names or share the identities of those who have made these excuses.)

Invite a volunteer to read 1 John 4:4; then discuss how this verse can encourage us when we are tempted. Relate David's sins to the fall of Adam and Eve, how he was tempted and his reaction after being caught in sin. Discuss the consequences of David's sin and the description of how his guilt affected him as recorded in Psalm 32. Bring the discussion around to the fact that guilt can affect our whole being and that it is only through confession of our sin that we can be healed of these effects.

Write the reference "Psalm 103" across the top of the flipchart or whiteboard. Ask group members to call out the descriptions of God and

His gracious actions as you write them under the heading. Keep the list visible until the close of the discussion time. Close in prayer, using the Psalm 103 list to praise God for His many attributes.

week six: don't tempt me!

Before the meeting begins, write on a poster board the three types of temptation (*the lust of the flesh, the lust of the eyes, the boastful pride of life*) from 1 John 2:16. Discuss how these relate to the temptations for Eve in Genesis. Discuss the question: "How can knowing the types of temptation help us when we feel the pull to give in to the temptations we encounter?"

Using the list, compare Jesus' temptations to the three types of temptations. Invite a volunteer to read Hebrews 2:17-18. Discuss how this passage is an encouragement to us as we are faced with temptation.

Have group members suggest examples of God's faithfulness as you record their answers on the flipchart or whiteboard. Discuss how knowing about God's faithfulness can encourage us in times of temptation. Invite volunteers to share how they have experienced God's faithfulness as they have resisted temptation. Ask members to share what encouragement they received from any Scripture from this week's lesson.

Invite a volunteer (or the whole group) to recite the Scripture memory verse for the week. Discuss the concept of temptation seizing us or dragging us down (see James 1:14). Help group members understand that we do have the power to resist and that resisting temptation leads to spiritual maturity.

Emphasize that we are to expect temptation, but that we can find a way out. Ask members to share ways that we can prepare to resist temptation and how we can flee the devil's schemes. Read Hebrews 4:15-16 as encouragement for the group. Remind them that our greatest weapons against the schemes of the devil are prayer and knowing God's Word.

Discuss how that when we do succumb to temptation, we might become defeated and want to give up, especially as it relates to trying to lose weight or attain a healthier lifestyle. Remind group members that God has given us a way to turn those feelings of defeat around. At those times of failure they can reach out to the Lord, repent and ask for forgiveness. Invite a member to read 1 John 1:9. Remind them to pray for one another throughout the week to be enabled to resist temptation.

week seven: a spiritual feast

Before class, prepare a display of various kinds of foods. On a tray, display a few examples of unhealthy junk foods. On another tray or in a bowl, display foods with good nutritional value. If possible, obtain a fresh unsliced loaf of multigrain bread to add to the display. Begin the discussion by relating the unhealthy food choices to the unhealthy choices we make in our lives. Then point out the beauty, smells and the nutritional value of the healthy foods. Compare the two types of foods to making wise choices in our lives and what the benefits of the good foods are.

Display the fresh loaf of bread. Discuss: "What do you think of when you smell bread? What does it mean for Jesus to be called the 'bread of life' and the 'bread come down from heaven'?" Lead the discussion so that members can experience the word pictures, comparing the aroma and beauty of the loaf of bread to the sweet aroma and beauty of those who follow Christ. Discuss how Jesus as the bread of life can encourage them to seek for the satisfaction that only comes from knowing Him.

Ask group members to look at the Day 3 chart and invite them to share their summaries, and then share their applications to these verses. As they share applications, write them on the flipchart or whiteboard. Discuss how these actions will help us grow as Christians. Invite a couple of volunteers to share an action they have taken during the week and the results of taking that action. Encourage others to take action toward savoring and eating God's Word.

Discuss the differences in the nutritional value of milk and solid food and how that relates to becoming spiritually mature. Ask what they would compare milk and solid food to in their spiritual walks. End the meeting by sharing the healthy foods with the group.

week eight: a new you

Before the meeting find a tight-fitting shirt, pair of pants or dress that you can barely squeeze into. You can either wear the item to the meeting or put it on in front of the class (it should be good for a few laughs as you squeeze into it). Wear this item of clothing while you lead the discussion.

An alternative visual aid would be to bring a stuffed animal and a clear plastic or glass container a little smaller than the animal. Proceed to stuff the toy into the container as you begin the meeting.

As you stuff either yourself or the toy animal, begin the discussion on the differences between being transformed and conformed. Ask for examples of how the world tries to conform us to its mold. Point out your discomfort of being squeezed into a mold that doesn't fit. Lead the discussion into an understanding that transformation takes time; it is not a quick fix for our problems, whereas conforming is usually easier because we merely imitate the actions of others.

Discuss the practical ways that the principles of Colossians 3:1-2,9-10 can be carried out in a believer's life. Ask members to share ways to renew their minds when negative thoughts or comments begin to take over.

Understanding God's will is not simple for even the most seasoned believers. Just when we think we've got it figured out, we learn something new. Help group members understand that the only way to really know God's will is to stay in close relationship with Him. Discuss what they learned from days 4 and 5 about God's will for their lives. Have them share about any Scripture verses that were especially meaningful as they studied about God's will.

As you complete this discussion time, pull, rip or cut off the item of too-tight clothing that you've been wearing (or release the poor little stuffed animal) and exclaim how good it feels to be freed from a mold that doesn't fit. Remind the group members that God's will for their lives is good, pleasing and perfect for each one of them.

week nine: the dwelling place of God

Before class, obtain a diagram of the Temple building. You might find one on the Internet, a Christian bookstore or your church's Sunday School materials. Attach the diagram to a piece of poster board.

Begin the meeting by reading Psalm 139 aloud. Those who struggle with weight or other physical problems may find it difficult to consider themselves "fearfully and wonderfully made." Help them see that God intended our bodies to work in harmony with the four-sided aspects of body, soul, mind and emotions and that when we achieve a balance in the four aspects, our bodies will work more in tune as God planned. Compare the animal sacrifices with being living sacrifices. Ask group members to share examples of being living sacrifices that honor God. Relate the discussion to Jesus as the once-for-all sacrifice for our sins.

On the diagram point out the various parts of the Temple as group members share what they know about the different parts of the building and the various functions of these parts. Discuss: "How does knowing that your body is God's temple affect your thinking about your own body? What new understanding have you come to concerning the significance of your body being the temple of God's Holy Spirit?" Also discuss the symbolism of the ripping of the veil as Jesus died on the cross—that it represents the opening of the Holy of Holies to all who believe.

Discuss the chart on the work of the Holy Spirit on Day 3. Invite volunteers to share a work of the Holy Spirit and how they will apply it to their lives. Also discuss how we might grieve the Holy Spirit and put out the Spirit's fire in our lives. Ask: "What can we do to get the relationship right again?"

Discuss ways we can honor God with our bodies. Guide the group to come up with concrete, practical ways and list them on the flipchart or whiteboard. Be sure to lead the discussion to include cheerful giving, giving to the needy and self-control. Remind the group that the mouth is part of the body. Ask someone to read James 3:3-10 and discuss how difficult it is to tame the tongue, but that we must in order to honor God.

Complete the discussion by sharing about how First Place 4 Health can teach us how to honor God with our whole being. Invite volunteers to share how First Place 4 Health has helped them. (*Note:* Next week's discussion asks for group members to bring an example of something that denotes success on the world's terms. If you plan to use this activity, give members the assignment before they leave.)

week ten: commit to the Lord

Before class, gather magazine, newspaper or TV advertisements that promote the world's definition of success. If possible, ask group members to each bring something that represents success on the world's terms.

Place the advertisements around the meeting room. Begin by asking group members how the examples illustrate worldly success. Invite volunteers to share how they would have defined success in their younger years and if any of those definitions have changed over the years. Have each person turn to a partner and share with one another their definition of God's view of success.

Before class, write on one page of the flipchart "What the Lord has done for me" and on another page write "What He asks of me." Attach these pages to the wall or board. Invite group members to share what the Lord has done for us as you write their responses on the chart, e.g., forgives us, died for us, loves us, protects us, etc. When you've completed that list, ask for their suggestions for what the Lord requires from us, e.g., commitment, faith, etc. Point out that the list of what the Lord has done for us is a lot longer than the list of what He requires of us.

Read 1 Samuel 7:3-4. Discuss what the foreign gods and Astoreths might be in our lives. Ask members to suggest some examples of what idols might be in our lives, pointing out that sometimes even good things can become idols. Then discuss how idols keep us from committing fully to God, distracting us from His plan.

Have group members point out some of the things that God did for the Israelites as listed in Psalm 78. Then have them share some of the rebellious acts that the people did. Point out the seriousness of rebelliousness and that there are consequences.

Have group members share what they learned about the rewards of a willing attitude toward God's commands. Invite volunteers to share about the delights they have experienced as they followed the Lord wholeheartedly. Discuss Matthew 11:28-30 and how this Scripture is related to First Place 4 Health goals.

week eleven: God is love!

Prepare large paper hearts cut out of red or pink construction paper. On seven of the paper hearts write the word "IS." On nine of the hearts "NOT." Write the corresponding words on the hearts from the chart on Day 1. Hand the hearts out to group members just before you begin the discussion. Ask each member holding a heart to read aloud what their heart says and give them a piece of tape to attach these to the walls around the room. Talk about how this kind of love only comes from God and how we can only successfully express this kind of love when we allow His Holy Spirit to express it through us in our actions and words.

Discuss the group members' answers to the last three questions on Day 1, asking group members to give specific examples of how these actions can be corrupted without love. (*Note*: The answers to the questions about the Hebrew words for "love" in Psalm 119: *hesed*—vv. 41,64,76; *'ahab*—vv. 47,48.)

Lead a discussion on the uniqueness of the command to "love one another." Discuss how this was not a command for believers to love unbelievers but for them to love *fellow believers*. Discuss why it is often hard to love fellow believers.

Discuss who else, besides fellow believers, we are supposed to love. Focus on the concept of loving enemies. Point out that Jews in Jesus' time felt that they could rightfully hate enemies, despite the fact that there is nowhere in the Old Testament that states it. It had just become a part of their traditions and manmade laws. Discuss: "How would the command to love one's enemies affect the Jews? How should it affect you?"

Discuss how sharing the gospel message is the ultimate act of love toward others. Invite a couple of volunteers to share their experiences of sharing Jesus with someone. Challenge the group members to share the ultimate gift of love with someone in the days and weeks to come.

week twelve: time to celebrate!

Even though most of your meeting this week will be a victory celebration, take time to talk about how much God loves us and how we are called to love our brothers and sisters in Christ because God loves us. (See "Planning a Victory Celebration" in the *First Place 4 Health Leader's Guide* for ideas about throwing a successful celebration for your group.)

During the past week, each member of your group will have prepared a *Seek God First* faith story. Spend time giving members an equal opportunity to share the good things God has done for them in this First Place 4 Health session. Make it clear that everyone should be given a chance to share at least a portion of his or her story. Don't allow the more talkative group members to monopolize all the time. Even the quiet members need an opportunity to share their stories! Be sure members share the progress they made, as reflected in the self-assessment done at the beginning of this Bible study.

End the victory celebration by having members offer up short sentence prayers of thanksgiving to the Lord for what He has accomplished for them during this session. Encourage even those who are shy about praying aloud in a group to pray at least a word or phrase of praise for what the Lord has done.

First Place 4 Health menu plans

Each menu plan is based on approximately 1,400 to 1,500 calories per day. All recipe and menu exchanges were determined using the Master-Cook software, a program that accesses a database containing more than 6,000 food items prepared using the United States Department of Agriculture (USDA) publications and information from food manufacturers. As with any nutritional program, MasterCook calculates the nutritional values of the recipes based on ingredients. Nutrition may vary due to how the food is prepared, where the food comes from, soil content, season, ripeness, processing and method of preparation. For these reasons, please use the recipes and menu plans as approximate guides. Consult a physician and/or a registered dietitian before starting a weight-loss program.

For those who need more calories, add the following to the 1,400-calorie plan:

- 1,800 calories: 2 ounce equivalent of meat, 3 ounce equivalent of bread, $1/2$ cup vegetable serving, 1 tsp. fat

- 2,000 calories: 2 ounce equivalent of meat, 4 ounce equivalent of bread, $1/2$ cup vegetable serving, 3 tsp. fat

- 2,200 calories: 2 ounce equivalent of meat, 5 ounce equivalent of bread, $1/2$ cup vegetable serving, $1/2$ cup fruit serving, 5 tsp. fat

- 2,400 calories: 2 ounce equivalent of meat, 6 ounce equivalent of bread, 1 cup vegetable serving, $1/2$ cup fruit serving, 6 tsp. fat

First Week Grocery List

Produce

- ☐ (1) bag green grapes
- ☐ (1) bag celery stalks
- ☐ (1) apple
- ☐ (2) plums
- ☐ (1) orange
- ☐ (1) peach
- ☐ (5) potatoes
- ☐ (1) banana
- ☐ $3/4$ cup blueberries
- ☐ (1) honeydew melon
- ☐ 1 cup raspberries
- ☐ (1) small mango
- ☐ 1 cup strawberries
- ☐ 4 cups snap beans
- ☐ (2) bunches broccoli
- ☐ (1) bunch cilantro
- ☐ $2^1/8$ tbsp. lime juice
- ☐ (4) jalapeno peppers
- ☐ (4) red onions
- ☐ (1) bunch spinach
- ☐ 2 cups green beans
- ☐ (4) Roma tomatoes
- ☐ (1) large tomato
- ☐ 1 cup mushrooms
- ☐ (11) garlic cloves
- ☐ (10) cherry tomatoes
- ☐ (1) bunch green onions
- ☐ (1) bunch dark green lettuce
- ☐ (1) cucumber
- ☐ (1) cantaloupe
- ☐ (1) bag carrots
- ☐ (1) bag carrot sticks
- ☐ $1/4$ cup fresh lemon juice

Breads and Cereals

- ☐ whole-wheat bread
- ☐ bagels
- ☐ whole-wheat English muffins
- ☐ (5) dinner rolls
- ☐ (6) breadsticks
- ☐ (1) pita bread
- ☐ (14) 6-inch low-fat tortillas
- ☐ (2) 16-ounce cans navy beans
- ☐ cornflakes
- ☐ fortified cereal of your choice
- ☐ wheat flake cereal
- ☐ saltine crackers
- ☐ brown rice

Canned Goods

- ☐ (1) 16-oz. can baked beans
- ☐ (1) 8-oz. can white meat chicken
- ☐ Healthy Choice® cream of chicken soup
- ☐ (2) 16-oz. cans low-sodium broth
- ☐ (1) can gazpacho soup
- ☐ (3) 4-oz. cans green chilies

Baking Products

- ☐ granulated sugar
- ☐ cooking wine
- ☐ cooking sherry
- ☐ flour
- ☐ marjoram
- ☐ Old Bay® seafood seasoning
- ☐ cinnamon
- ☐ dried thyme
- ☐ dried onions

- ❑ paprika
- ❑ dried parsley
- ❑ lemon pepper seasoning
- ❑ cayenne pepper
- ❑ bay leaves
- ❑ Creole seasoning
- ❑ salt
- ❑ pepper
- ❑ dried oregano
- ❑ ground cumin
- ❑ Dijon mustard
- ❑ Worcestershire sauce
- ❑ vegetable oil or canola oil
- ❑ olive oil
- ❑ low-fat mayonnaise
- ❑ chunky-style spaghetti sauce
- ❑ BBQ sauce
- ❑ reduced-calorie maple-flavored syrup
- ❑ orange marmalade
- ❑ $1/4$ cup salsa
- ❑ low-sodium soy sauce

Dairy Products

- ❑ 4 oz. reduced-fat Colby-Jack cheese
- ❑ 20 oz. low-fat cheddar cheese
- ❑ 2 oz. low-fat mozzarella cheese
- ❑ nonfat milk
- ❑ light margarine
- ❑ 32 oz. nonfat plain yogurt
- ❑ 10 oz. light sour cream

Seafood and Meat

- ❑ $1^1/_2$ lbs. cod
- ❑ $1/4$ lb. shrimp
- ❑ $1/2$ lb. catfish
- ❑ 1 oz. turkey bacon
- ❑ 1 oz. turkey pepperoni
- ❑ (1) reduced-fat hot dog
- ❑ low-fat Italian turkey sausage
- ❑ $2^1/_2$ lbs. skinless, boneless chicken breasts

Frozen Foods

- ❑ frozen whole-wheat waffles
- ❑ $2^1/_2$ cups frozen corn kernels
- ❑ $1/2$ cup frozen broccoli florets

First Week Meals and Recipes

DAY 1

Breakfast

2 whole-wheat frozen waffles
1 tsp. light margarine
1 cup nonfat milk

2 tsp. reduced-calorie maple syrup
1 cup honeydew melon

Nutritional Information: 502 calories (12% calories from fat); 2g fat; 9g protein; 32g carbohydrate; 1g dietary fiber; 4mg cholesterol; 208mg sodium; 313mg calcium.

Lunch

Veggie Cheese Quesadillas
nonstick cooking spray
2 oz. reduced-fat Colby-Jack cheese,
  grated
1/4 cup mushrooms, sliced

2 (6-inch) nonfat tortillas
1 tbsp. reduced-fat sour cream
1/2 cup frozen broccoli florets, cooked
1/4 cup salsa

Coat a nonstick skillet with cooking spray and heat. Put one tortilla in pan and sprinkle with cheese. Place broccoli and mushrooms on top of cheese. Cover with the second tortilla and brown on both sides. Remove from pan and let sit a minute. Slice and serve with sour cream and salsa. Serve with 1 cup carrot sticks and 1/2 cup sliced peaches in own juice.

Nutritional Information: 458 calories (13% calories from fat); 7g fat; 26g protein; 79g carbohydrate; 24g dietary fiber; 15mg cholesterol; 1,077mg sodium; 425mg calcium; 4mg iron.

Dinner

Grilled Chicken Breasts with Corn Salsa
Salsa
1 1/2 cups frozen corn kernels, thawed
1/4 cup red bell pepper, chopped
1 1/2 tbsp. fresh lime juice

1/4 cup red onion, chopped
1/4 cup fresh cilantro, chopped

Combine all ingredients in bowl. Season with salt and pepper. May be made the day before; cover and refrigerate.

Chicken
1/2 cup cooking sherry
1 tbsp. fresh cilantro, chopped
1 to 2 tsp. (to taste) jalapenos,
  chopped and seeded

1 tbsp. low-sodium soy sauce
2 tsp. fresh lime juice
4 skinless, boneless chicken breast halves

Combine first five ingredients in medium bowl. Add chicken and turn to coat. Cover and refrigerate at least 1 hour or up to 4 hours. Preheat barbecue (medium-high heat) or broiler. Drain chicken; season with salt and pepper to taste. Grill or broil chicken until cooked through, about 4 minutes per side. Cut chicken into thin diagonal slices. Arrange chicken on plates. Top with salsa and serve. Serve with spinach salad with sliced mushrooms and tomatoes, 1 cup cooked green beans mixed with a little salsa and a dinner roll with 1 tsp. reduced-calorie margarine per person.

Nutritional Information: 412 calories (10% calories from fat); 4g fat; 59g protein; 27g carbohydrate; 4g dietary fiber; 137mg cholesterol; 362mg sodium; 74mg calcium; 4mg iron.

DAY 2

....

Breakfast

1 small (2 oz.) whole-wheat English muffin, split and toasted
1 cup nonfat milk

1 tsp. light margarine
1 cup strawberries, sliced

Nutritional Information: 290 calories (13% calories from fat); 4g fat; 15g protein; 50g carbohydrate; 8g dietary fiber; 4mg cholesterol; 594mg sodium; 501mg calcium; 2 mg iron.

....

Lunch

Soup and Salad
1 serving of canned gazpacho
2 plums

2 (1-oz.) breadsticks, topped with 2 oz. reduced-fat Colby-Jack cheese, shredded

Nutritional Information: 451 calories (21% calories from fat); 10g fat; 29g protein; 61g carbohydrate; 2g dietary fiber; 12mg cholesterol; 1,459mg sodium; 277 calcium; 2mg iron.

....

Dinner

Spicy White Bean and Chicken Chili
2 cans (16-oz.) navy beans
1 extra-large onion, chopped
$1/2$ tsp. dried oregano, crumbled
$3/4$ lb. boneless, skinless chicken breast, well-trimmed, cut in large pieces
$3/4$ cup plain nonfat yogurt
3 jalapenos, minced (optional)
2 cans (4-oz.) green chilies, diced

2 tsp. olive oil
8 large garlic cloves, minced
$5^1/4$ cups canned unsalted chicken broth
fresh cilantro, chopped
1 tbsp. ground cumin
$3/4$ cup water

Heat oil in large, heavy pot over medium heat. Add onion and garlic and sauté until tender, about 10 minutes. Stir in cumin and oregano and cook 1 minute. Mix in beans and chilies, then chicken, broth and water. Simmer until beans are very tender and chili is creamy, about 1 hour and 45 minutes or less. (*Note:* May be made 3 days ahead. Cover and refrigerate. Reheat when ready to serve.) Ladle chili into bowls. Garnish with yogurt, cilantro and minced chilies and serve immediately. Serve with a spinach salad with reduced-calorie dressing. Serves 4.

Nutritional Information: 549 calories (23% calories from fat); 16g fat; 57g protein; 62g carbohydrate; 13g dietary fiber; 1mg cholesterol; 1,109mg sodium; 287mg calcium; 9mg iron.

DAY 3

Breakfast

1 cup fortified cold cereal $^1/_2$ small mango
1 cup nonfat milk

Nutritional Information: 263 calories (6% calories from fat); 2g fat; 12g protein; 53g carbohydrate; 5g dietary fiber; 4mg cholesterol; 348mg sodium; 313mg calcium.

Lunch

Chicken Patty Melt
2 slices whole-wheat bread   1 oz. canned white chicken meat
2 tsp. reduced-fat mayonnaise   1 oz. shredded part-skim mozzarella
                                      cheese

Toast bread. Combine chicken, mayonnaise and cheese in small bowl, and spread on toasted bread. Broil open-faced until bubbly. Serve with 1 cup of celery sticks, 1 tbsp. fat-free Ranch dressing and 1 medium apple.

Nutritional Information: 477 calories (25% calories from fat); 14g fat; 23g protein; 69g carbohydrate; 12g dietary fiber; 36mg cholesterol; 1,041mg sodium; 331mg calcium; 4mg iron.

Dinner

Lite Chicken Enchiladas
1 (8 oz.) container light sour cream   1 (4 oz.) can green chilies, diced
1 ($10^1/_2$ oz.) can Healthy Choice cream   12 (6-inch) low-fat tortillas
  of chicken soup
$1^1/_2$ cups cooked chicken, chopped   1 (8 oz.) container plain nonfat yogurt
1 cup reduced-fat cheddar cheese, $^1/_4$ cup green onions, sliced
  shredded
nonstick cooking spray

Heat oven to 350° F. Spray a 13x9-inch (3-quart) baking dish with cooking spray. In medium bowl, combine sour cream, yogurt, soup and chilies, mix well. Spoon about 3 tbsp. sour cream mixture down the center of each tortilla. Reserve $^1/_4$ cup of cheddar cheese; sprinkle each tortilla with remaining cheese, chicken and onions. Roll tortillas and place in spray-coated dish, seam side down. Spoon remaining sour-cream mixture over tortillas. Cover with foil and bake 25 to 30 minutes, or until hot and bubbly. Remove foil, sprinkle with reserved $^1/_4$ cup cheese. Return to oven uncovered and bake an additional 5 minutes or until cheese is melted. Serve enchiladas on top of shredded lettuce and chopped tomatoes with $^1/_2$ cup salsa per person. Serves 6.

Nutritional Information: 743 calories (23% calories from fat); 19g fat; 49g protein; 95g carbohydrate; 7g dietary fiber; 68mg cholesterol; 2,173mg sodium; 477mg calcium; 5mg iron.

DAY 4

Breakfast
1 slice whole-wheat bread, toasted and topped with 1 tsp. light margarine and
 $^1/_2$ tsp. granulated sugar and pinch of cinnamon
$^3/_4$ cup nonfat plain vanilla yogurt mixed with $^3/_4$ cup blueberries

Nutritional Information: 319 calories (13% calories from fat); 5g fat; 16g protein; 56g carbohydrate; 7g dietary fiber; 3mg cholesterol; 478mg sodium; 388mg calcium; 2mg iron.

Lunch

Veggie Pizza
1 (6-inch) flat pita bread
$^1/_4$ cup broccoli florets
$^1/_4$ cup prepared chunky-style spaghetti sauce
1 oz. part-skim mozzarella, shredded

$^1/_4$ cup carrots, shredded
$^1/_4$ cup tomatoes, diced
8 turkey pepperoni slices

Preheat oven to 450° F. Place pita bread on a cookie sheet. Spread sauce on top of bread. Layer with remaining ingredients, finishing with the cheese. Bake 8 to 10 minutes or until cheese is melted and bubbly. Serve with 1 small orange.

Nutritional Information: 477 calories (24% calories from fat); 13g fat; 25g protein; 66g carbohydrate; 9g dietary fiber; 53mg cholesterol; 1,368mg sodium; 348mg calcium; 3mg iron.

Dinner

Quick Baked Fish
$1^1/_2$ lbs. cod, tilapia, catfish or haddock fillets
2 tsp. dried onion flakes
1 tsp. Old Bay seasoning

$^1/_4$ cup low-fat mayonnaise
1 tsp. Dijon mustard
1 tsp. white wine Worcestershire sauce
$^1/_4$ tsp. paprika

1 tbsp. dried (or 2 tbsp. fresh, chopped) $1/2$ tsp. lemon pepper
  parsley   nonstick cooking spray
$1/8$ tsp. cayenne pepper

Preheat oven to 400° F. Spray a shallow casserole dish with cooking spray; set aside. Wash fillets with cold water and pat dry with paper towels. Place fish fillets in prepared dish. In a small bowl, combine remaining ingredients until well mixed. Spread mixture evenly over fillets. Bake uncovered for 15 minutes or until fish flakes easily with a fork. Serve with steamed broccoli and $1/2$ cup cooked brown rice and one breadstick per person. Serves 4.

Nutritional Information: 431 calories (21% calories from fat); 12g fat; 39g protein; 58g carbohydrate; 7g dietary fiber; 104mg cholesterol; 644mg sodium; 116mg calcium; 3mg iron.

DAY 5

Breakfast

$3/4$ cup corn flakes $1/2$ medium banana, sliced
1 cup nonfat milk

Nutritional Information: 293 calories (3% calories from fat); 1g fat; 12g protein; 62g carbohydrate; 3g dietary fiber; 4mg cholesterol; 574mg sodium; 308mg calcium; 13mg iron.

Lunch

BBQ Franks and Beans
1 reduced-fat, all-beef frank, diced   1 cup baked beans, drained
1 tbsp. prepared BBQ sauce

Combine all ingredients. Microwave for 2 to 3 minutes. Serve with 1 cup cantaloupe cubes, and 1 cup peeled and sliced cucumber tossed with 1 tbsp. light Italian dressing.

Nutritional Information: 430 calories (6% calories from fat); 3g fat; 19g protein; 95g carbohydrate; 18g dietary fiber; 0mg cholesterol; 1,349mg sodium; 198 mg calcium; 3mg iron.

Dinner

Marmalade Chicken
$1/4$ cup orange marmalade $1/4$ cup fresh lemon juice
$1/4$ cup white cooking wine   1 tbsp. soy sauce, diluted with 1 tbsp. water
$1/4$ tsp. dried thyme, crumbled   1 (3-lb.) chicken, cut into 4 pieces

Combine first 5 ingredients in large bowl. Remove any visible fat from chicken, but leave skin on. Add chicken to bowl with marinade; toss to coat. Cover and refrigerate 4 hours or overnight, stirring occasionally. Preheat oven to 400° F.

Place a wire rack on top of a baking sheet. Remove chicken from marinade, reserving marinade. Place chicken skin-side up on rack. Bake 20 minutes. Turn and bake 20 minutes longer. Turn chicken skin-side up and continue cooking until skin is golden brown and chicken is almost cooked through, approximately 10 minutes. Meanwhile, boil marinade in small, heavy saucepan until reduced to glaze, about 10 minutes. Remove skin and brush chicken with glaze. Bake chicken until glaze is set and chicken is cooked through, approximately 5 minutes. Serve with 1 cup roasted potatoes, 1 cup sautéed snap peas and 1 dinner roll per person. Serves 4.

Nutritional Information: 573 calories (6% calories from fat); 4g fat; 38g protein; 96g carbohydrate; 11g dietary fiber; 69mg cholesterol; 525mg sodium; 143mg calcium; 7mg iron.

DAY 6

Breakfast

1 small (2 oz.) bagel, toasted and topped with 1 tsp. light margarine
$3/4$ cup raspberries
1 cup nonfat milk

Nutritional Information: 287 calories (11% calories from fat); 4g fat; 14g protein; 50g carbohydrate; 10g dietary fiber; 4mg cholesterol; 410mg sodium; 364mg calcium; 2mg iron.

Lunch

Stuffed Potato

1 (6-oz.) potato, baked
$1/4$ cup tomato, diced
1 tsp. light margarine
$1/4$ cup cooked broccoli florets
1 tbsp. fat-free sour cream

1 oz. turkey bacon, cooked and crumbled
1 tbsp. green onions, diced
1 oz. reduced-fat cheddar cheese, shredded
$1/4$ cup mushrooms, sliced

Slice open the baked potato and scoop out insides into a small bowl. Combine with remaining ingredients and mix well. Fill shell with the mixture. Microwave until hot. Serve with 15 grapes.

Nutritional Information: 392 calories (22% calories from fat); 10g fat; 19g protein; 61g carbohydrate; 7g dietary fiber; 33mg cholesterol; 628mg sodium; 214mg calcium; 2mg iron.

Dinner

Argentine Corn Chicken

1 lb. boneless chicken breasts, skinless, cut into chunks
$1/4$ tsp. leaf marjoram

2 cloves garlic, minced
pepper, freshly ground, to taste
$1/2$ medium onion, chopped

1 tbsp. canola oil
10 whole cherry tomatoes
1 bay leaf

1 large tomato, seeded, chopped
1 cup frozen whole-kernel corn, thawed
salt

Season chicken lightly with salt and pepper. In a large nonstick skillet, heat oil. Add chicken and cook until tender, turning occasionally to prevent burning. Remove from skillet and set aside; keep warm. Sauté onion and garlic in skillet. Add chopped tomato, bay leaf and marjoram; simmer 10 minutes. Add corn, whole cherry tomatoes and chicken to skillet and heat through, mixing well. Serve each with $1/3$ cup brown rice and 1 cup steamed vegetables. Serves 4.

Nutritional Information: 426 calories (35% calories from fat); 17g fat; 36g protein; 37g carbohydrate; 8g dietary fiber; 0mg cholesterol; 50mg sodium.

DAY 7

Breakfast

1 cup fortified cold cereal
1 cup nonfat milk

$1/2$ medium banana, sliced

Nutritional Information: 254 calories (9% calories from fat); 2g fat; 12g protein; 49g carbohydrate; 4g dietary fiber; 4mg cholesterol; 411mg sodium; calcium 361mg; 8mg iron.

Lunch

McDonald's® Happy Meal™
Diet soda

Tossed green salad with fat-free salad dressing

Nutritional Information: 524 calories (38% calories from fat); 22g fat; 18g protein; 65g carbohydrate; 8g dietary fiber; 25mg cholesterol; 673mg sodium; 169mg calcium; 2mg iron.

Dinner

Seafood and Turkey Sausage Gumbo
$1/4$ cup all-purpose flour
3 garlic cloves, chopped
1 cup canned low-salt chicken or
   vegetable broth
$1/4$ pound small shrimp, de-veined
1 cup green bell pepper, chopped
10-oz. low-fat Italian turkey sausages,
   casings removed

1 cup chopped onion
1 bay leaf
1 can (28-oz.) tomatoes in juice, diced
1 tbsp. vegetable oil
1 tsp. dried thyme
2 tsp. Creole or Cajun seasoning
2 (4-oz.) catfish fillets, each cut
   into 4 pieces

Sprinkle flour over bottom of heavy, large pot. Stir flour constantly over medium-low heat until flour turns golden brown (do not allow to burn), about 12 to 15 minutes. Pour browned flour into bowl, set aside. Heat oil in same pot over medium heat. Add onion and bell pepper; stir 1 minute. Add sausages and sauté until brown, breaking up with back of spoon, about 5 minutes. Add browned flour. Add tomatoes with juice, broth and Creole seasoning. Bring to boil. Reduce heat, cover and simmer 20 minutes to blend flavors, stirring frequently. Add shrimp and catfish to pot and simmer until seafood is opaque in center, about 5 minutes. Discard bay leaf. Season with salt and pepper and serve. Serve over $1/2$ cup steamed brown rice and with a green salad mixed with 2 tbsp. reduced-fat dressing and 4 saltine crackers for each person. Serves 4.

Nutritional Information: 589 calories (33.9% calories from fat); 23g fat; 37g protein; 62g carbohydrate; 7g dietary fiber; 132mg cholesterol; 1,091mg sodium; 172mg calcium; 6 mg iron.

Second Week Grocery List

Produce
- ❑ (1) peach
- ❑ ³/₄ cup blueberries
- ❑ ³/₄ cup blackberries
- ❑ 2 cups strawberries
- ❑ (1) grapefruit
- ❑ (1) onion
- ❑ (9) garlic cloves
- ❑ (1) green pepper
- ❑ (1) bag carrots
- ❑ (1) package fresh parsley
- ❑ 3 lbs. snap peas
- ❑ (2) bags green grapes
- ❑ (1) bunch cilantro
- ❑ 1 tbsp. fresh lime juice
- ❑ (1) jalapeno
- ❑ (1) head cabbage
- ❑ 1 lb. mushrooms
- ❑ (1) bunch green onions
- ❑ (1) bunch green cabbage leaves
- ❑ fresh basil
- ❑ fresh ginger
- ❑ fresh rosemary
- ❑ fresh sage
- ❑ (1) red bell pepper
- ❑ (2) red onions
- ❑ (1) zucchini
- ❑ (1) small eggplant
- ❑ 2 tsp. fresh lemon juice
- ❑ (1) bunch broccoli
- ❑ (4) potatoes
- ❑ (1) bunch celery
- ❑ (1) large cucumber
- ❑ (1) bag baby carrots
- ❑ (1) package alfalfa sprouts
- ❑ (1) bag mixed salad greens
- ❑ (1) bunch cauliflower
- ❑ (2) apples
- ❑ (1) bunch spinach
- ❑ (2) tomatoes

Baking Products
- ❑ cooking spray
- ❑ brown sugar
- ❑ cooking wine
- ❑ Worcestershire sauce
- ❑ Dijon mustard
- ❑ mustard
- ❑ canola oil
- ❑ olive oil
- ❑ sesame oil
- ❑ sesame seeds
- ❑ low-sodium soy sauce
- ❑ teriyaki sauce
- ❑ sugar substitute
- ❑ salt
- ❑ pepper
- ❑ ground cumin
- ❑ coarse salt
- ❑ (3) cloves
- ❑ lemon pepper seasoning
- ❑ rice wine vinegar
- ❑ balsamic vinegar
- ❑ brown rice
- ❑ raisins
- ❑ strawberry jam
- ❑ all-purpose flour
- ❑ Chinese noodles
- ❑ reduced-fat mayonnaise
- ❑ low-calorie Thousand Island dressing

- ❏ reduced-fat salad dressing
- ❏ low-calorie maple syrup

Breads and Cereals
- ❏ whole-wheat bread
- ❏ English muffins
- ❏ small bagels
- ❏ sourdough bread
- ❏ whole-wheat pita bread
- ❏ French bread
- ❏ rye bread
- ❏ wheat flakes cereal
- ❏ bran flakes
- ❏ raisin bran
- ❏ (6) low-fat 7-inch flour tortillas
- ❏ saltine crackers

Canned Foods
- ❏ (1) can fruit cocktail in juice
- ❏ (1) can pineapple chunks
- ❏ (1) can tuna in water
- ❏ (1) can tomatoes
- ❏ (1) can sauerkraut
- ❏ (1) can mixed vegetables
- ❏ (1) can Mandarin oranges
- ❏ (2) cans chicken broth
- ❏ (1) can beef broth

Dairy Products
- ❏ reduced-fat cheddar cheese
- ❏ 6 oz. reduced-fat Swiss cheese
- ❏ reduced-fat Monterey-Jack cheese
- ❏ nonfat milk
- ❏ light margarine
- ❏ 20 oz. nonfat plain yogurt
- ❏ light sour cream

Seafood and Meat
- ❏ 1 lb. large fresh uncooked shrimp
- ❏ 2 oz. sliced lean roast beef
- ❏ 2 lbs. sirloin steaks, trimmed
- ❏ 12 oz. 98% fat-free smoked turkey
- ❏ $1^1/_4$ lbs. boneless skinless chicken breasts
- ❏ 4 skinless chicken breasts (bone-in)
- ❏ $1^1/_2$ oz. corned beef
- ❏ 2 oz. cooked turkey breast

Frozen Foods
- ❏ (1) 11-oz. lean frozen dinner entrée
- ❏ Lean Cuisine® Pasta Alfredo frozen pancakes
- ❏ 4 cups Oriental vegetables

Second Week Meals and Recipes

DAY 1

Breakfast

2 slices sourdough bread, toasted and topped with1 tsp. light margarine
3/4 cup blueberries
1 cup nonfat milk

Nutritional Information: 304 calories (12% calories from fat); 4g fat; 13g protein; 53g carbohydrate; 4g dietary fiber; 4mg cholesterol; 483mg sodium; 347mg calcium; 2mg iron.

Lunch

Chef's Salad

1 cup dark, mixed salad greens
1 cup vegetables (broccoli, carrots,
  zucchini, onion, cauliflower,
  bell pepper), chopped
1 oz. reduced-fat Swiss cheese, diced
1 oz. cooked turkey, diced

3/4 cup Mandarin oranges
1 tbsp. reduced-fat dressing
8 saltines

Combine first five ingredients and toss in reduced-fat dressing.

Nutritional Information: 410 calories (23.1% calories from fat); 10g fat; 24g protein; 55g carbohydrate; 14g dietary fiber; 31mg cholesterol; 1,164mg sodium; 438mg calcium; 4mg iron.

Dinner

Smoked Turkey Quesadillas

nonstick cooking spray
12 oz. 98% fat-free smoked turkey, sliced
6 (7-inch) low-fat tortillas
fresh cilantro sprigs, stemmed
coarse salt

6 oz. low-fat Monterey-Jack cheese, grated
1/2 tsp. ground cumin
36 green grapes, halved lengthwise
1 tbsp. fresh lime juice

Place tortillas on work surface. Arrange cheese, turkey, grapes and cilantro over half of each tortilla. Sprinkle with cumin. Fold tortillas over filling. Preheat oven to 200° F. Heat large, nonstick skillet over medium heat. Coat with vegetable spray. Cook quesadillas, one at a time, until golden brown, about 3 minutes, turning once. Turn again. Brush cooked top with lime juice and sprinkle with coarse salt. Cook until golden brown, about 3 minutes. Keep warm in oven. Repeat with remaining quesadillas. Serve each with 1/4 cup chunky salsa mixed with 1 tsp. reduced-fat sour cream. Serves 6.

Nutritional Information: 483 calories (25% calories from fat); 13g fat; 24g protein; 63g carbohydrate; 5g dietary fiber; 20mg cholesterol; 888mg sodium; 650mg calcium.

DAY 2

Breakfast

1 small (2 oz.) bagel, toasted and topped with 1 tsp. strawberry jam
3/4 cup artificially sweetened mixed-berry nonfat yogurt, mixed with
    3/4 cup blackberries

Nutritional Information: 310 calories (5% calories from fat); 2g fat; 16g protein; 59g carbohydrate; 7g dietary fiber; 3mg cholesterol; 409mg sodium; 413mg calcium; 3mg iron.

Lunch

Sandwich and Salad

2 slices whole-grain bread
2 oz. cooked turkey breast, sliced

1 tsp. reduced-fat mayonnaise
mustard and pickle (optional)

Serve with tossed green salad mixed with sliced tomatoes, cucumbers, carrots and peppers, 2 tbsp. fat-free salad dressing and 1/3 cup pineapple tidbits.

Nutritional Information: 374 calories (13% calories from fat); 6g fat; 25g protein; 61g carbohydrate; 10g dietary fiber; 39mg cholesterol; 554mg sodium; 156mg calcium; 6mg iron.

Dinner

Rosemary-Sage Steak

1 lb. boneless top sirloin steak, all visible fat removed

Marinade

1/2 cup onion, chopped
1 tsp. olive oil
2 tbsp. fresh (or 2 tsp. dried,
   crushed) rosemary, finely chopped
2 tbsp. fresh (or 2 tsp. dried, crushed)
   sage, finely chopped
3 medium cloves garlic, minced
   (or 1 1/2 tsp. bottled, minced)

3 tbsp. dry white cooking wine
1/4 tsp. salt
1/4 cup fresh lemon juice
1 tbsp. Dijon mustard
1/2 tsp. pepper

Put steak in an airtight plastic bag. In a small bowl, combine marinade ingredients. Pour into bag over steak and turn to coat evenly. Seal and refrigerate from 1 to 24 hours, turning occasionally. Preheat grill on medium-high heat. Drain steak; grill for 8 to 12 minutes per side, or until done to taste. Serve with

1 cup grilled vegetables, and a 6-ounce potato topped with 1 tsp. reduced-calorie margarine and 1 tsp. reduced-fat sour cream per person. Serves 4.

Nutritional Information: 418 calories (21% calories from fat); 10g fat; 33g protein; 52g carbohydrate; 11g dietary fiber; 67mg cholesterol; 362mg sodium; 161mg calcium; 6mg iron.

DAY 3

Breakfast

1 small (2 oz.) English muffin, toasted and topped with 1 tsp. light margarine
$1/_2$ medium grapefruit
1 cup nonfat milk

Nutritional Information. 278 calories (11% calories from fat); 3g fat; 13g protein; 48g carbohydrate; 3g dietary fiber; 4mg cholesterol; 435mg sodium; 416mg calcium; 2mg iron.

Lunch

11 oz. lean frozen dinner entrée   1 cup fresh baby carrots
1 small apple

Nutritional Information: 424 calories (16% calories from fat); 8g fat; 20g protein; 70g carbohydrate; 9g dietary fiber; 30mg cholesterol; 711mg sodium; 273mg calcium; 1mg iron.

Dinner

Grilled Sesame Chicken
2 tbsp. sesame seeds
$1/_4$ tsp. black pepper, freshly ground
2 tbsp. soy sauce, diluted with $1^1/_2$ tbsp. water
3 cloves garlic, crushed
1 tbsp. brown sugar
4 (3-oz.) uncooked skinless chicken breasts

Combine first five ingredients in a shallow dish. Mix well. Add chicken, turning to coat. Cover and refrigerate for at least 2 hours. Remove chicken from marinade. Grill 4 to 5 inches from medium-hot coals for 15 minutes. Turn and grill until done. Serve with 1 cup cooked noodles tossed with 1 tsp. teriyaki sauce and 1 cup sautéed Oriental vegetables per person.

Nutritional Information: 419 calories (11% calories from fat); 5g fat; 40g protein; 53g carbohydrate; 7g dietary fiber; 68mg cholesterol; 865mg sodium; 148mg calcium; 6mg iron.

DAY 4

Breakfast

1 cup wheat flakes cereal   1 medium peach, sliced
1 cup nonfat milk

Nutritional Information: 242 calories (6% calories from fat); 2g fat; 12g protein; 47g carbohydrate; 5g dietary fiber; 4mg cholesterol; 346mg sodium; 307mg calcium.

Lunch

French-Dip Roast Beef Sandwich
1 (4 oz.) loaf French bread
2 oz. lean, boneless roast beef, cooked and thinly sliced
1 cup hot, low-sodium beef broth

Cut bread loaf in half horizontally, and then cut pieces in half vertically to make 4 pieces. Place 2 of the pieces, cut side up, on each of 2 plates. Top each bread piece with 1 oz. roast beef and $^1/_4$ cup broth. Cover each plate with plastic wrap; microwave for 30 to 45 seconds until heated through. Serve with 1 cup broccoli florets with 2 tbsp. reduced-fat Ranch dressing and 1 cup strawberries per person. Serves 2.

Nutritional Information: 388 calories (16% calories from fat); 6g fat; 21g protein; 45g carbohydrate; 10g dietary fiber; 31mg cholesterol; 667mg sodium; 133mg calcium; 3mg iron.

Dinner

Shrimp Scampi
1 lb. large fresh uncooked shrimp,   1 tsp. olive oil
   de-veined   1 tsp. margarine, melted
1 clove garlic, minced   1 tbsp. fresh parsley, chopped
$^1/_4$ tsp. black pepper, freshly ground
$^1/_4$ cup white cooking wine

Combine margarine, oil, garlic, cooking wine and pepper in a large bowl. Add shrimp and toss lightly to coat. Spread a single layer of shrimp in a shallow, oven-safe casserole dish. Broil shrimp approximately 4 inches from heat for 3 to 4 minutes. Turn shrimp and broil for an additional 3 to 4 minutes or until lightly browned. Sprinkle with fresh chopped parsley and serve. Serve with Lean Cuisine Pasta Alfredo and snap peas. Serves 4.

Nutritional Information: 504 calories (38.4% calories from fat); 12g fat; 31g protein; 12g carbohydrate; 6g dietary fiber; 215mg cholesterol; 235mg sodium; 336mg calcium; 2mg iron.

DAY 5

Breakfast

$^3/_4$ cup bran flakes cereal   2 tbsp. raisins
1 cup nonfat milk

Nutritional Information: 277 calories (5% calories from fat); 2g fat; 13g protein; 56g carbohydrate; 4g dietary fiber; 4mg cholesterol; 403mg sodium; 311mg calcium.

Lunch

Tuna Salad Pita

4 oz. water-packed tuna, drained   2 tbsp. reduced-calorie mayonnaise
$^1/_4$ cup celery, chopped   1 (2-oz.) whole-wheat pita
$^1/_4$ tsp. lemon pepper seasoning $^1/_2$ cup alfalfa sprouts
$^1/_4$ cup onion, chopped

In a small bowl, combine first five ingredients. Cut one large whole-wheat pita in half crosswise and open to form two pockets. Fill each pocket with half the tuna salad and top each portion with $^1/_4$ cup alfalfa sprouts. Serve with 1 cup cucumber rounds, 1 cup carrot sticks and 15 grapes.

Nutritional Information: 388 calories (16% calories from fat); 6g fat; 22g protein; 51g carbohydrate; 9g dietary fiber; 22mg cholesterol; 516mg sodium; 84mg calcium; 3mg iron.

Dinner

Green Pepper Steak

1 lb. lean sirloin steak, cut into   2 tbsp. all-purpose flour
   $^1/_4$-inch strips   1 can beef broth
$^1/_4$ tsp. pepper, freshly ground $^1/_2$ tsp. salt
1 medium onion, sliced   1 cup canned tomatoes with juice
1 tbsp. canola oil $1^1/_2$ tsp. Worcestershire sauce
1 clove garlic, finely chopped
1 large green pepper, cut in strips

Coat strips of round steak with flour mixed with salt and pepper. Heat oil in a large frying pan. Brown meat on all sides; drain off any fat. Add broth, tomato juice (reserving tomato pieces), onion and garlic to meat. Cover and simmer about 30 to 40 minutes or until meat is tender. Add tomato pieces, green pepper strips and Worcestershire sauce. Stir and cook 10 minutes longer. Serve over $^1/_2$ cup cooked brown rice and with $^1/_2$ cup cooked carrots per person. Serves 4.

Nutritional Information: 476 calories (37% calories from fat); 20g fat; 29g protein; 45g carbohydrate; 5g dietary fiber; 71mg cholesterol; 806mg sodium; 78mg calcium; 4mg iron.

DAY 6

Breakfast

3 frozen pancakes, heated and topped with 2 tsp. low-calorie maple syrup
$1/2$ medium grapefruit
1 cup nonfat milk

Nutritional Information: 410 calories (9% calories from fat); 3g fat; 15g protein; 63g carbohydrate; 3g dietary fiber; 18mg cholesterol; 842mg sodium; 412mg calcium; 1mg iron.

Lunch

Waldorf Salad with Cheese

1 small apple, cored and diced
$1/2$ cup celery, chopped
2 cups red cabbage, shredded

2 oz. reduced-fat cheddar cheese, grated
2 tsp. reduced-calorie mayonnaise

In medium bowl, combine apple, celery, cheese and mayonnaise. Top shredded cabbage with salad mixture. Serve with 4 graham crackers ($2^1/2$–inch squares).

Nutritional Information: 382 calories (23.7% calories from fat); 11g fat; 19g protein; 57g carbohydrate; 9g dietary fiber; 15mg cholesterol; 635mg sodium; 366mg calcium; 3mg iron.

Dinner

Roasted Vegetable Sandwiches

8 slices sourdough bread or 4 pocket pita bread or 4 (2-oz.) rolls
4 oz. low-fat Swiss cheese, sliced

Basil-Yogurt Spread
$1/4$ cup plain nonfat yogurt
2 tbsp. reduced-fat mayonnaise

1 tbsp. fresh basil
1 tsp. lemon juice

Whisk together ingredients (can be prepared ahead and refrigerated).

Roasted Vegetables
3 tbsp. balsamic or red wine vinegar
$1/4$ cup fresh (or 1 tbsp. dried) basil, chopped
1 red bell pepper, seeded, thinly sliced
1 zucchini, thinly sliced

2 tsp. olive oil
1 yellow summer squash, thinly sliced
1 small red onion, sliced and separated
1 small eggplant, sliced into thin rounds

Preheat oven to 450° F. Blend vinegar, oil and basil. Add vegetables, tossing to coat. Place vegetables in roasting pan and cook, stirring occasionally, until tender and lightly browned, about 30 minutes. Cool vegetables. To assemble sandwiches, spread basil-yogurt mixture on your favorite bread, pita halves or crusty rolls. Top with cheese, fill with veggie mixture and serve. Serves 4.

Nutritional Information: 304 calories (22% calories from fat); 8g fat; 16g protein; 45g carbohydrate; 7g dietary fiber; 13mg cholesterol; 432mg sodium; 377mg calcium; 2mg iron.

DAY 7

Breakfast

$3/4$ cup raisin-bran cereal
1 cup nonfat milk
1 cup strawberries, sliced

1 slice reduced calorie wheat bread,
   toasted and topped with
1 tsp. light margarine

Nutritional Information: 336 calories (12% calories from fat); 5g fat; 16g protein; 64g carbohydrate; 10g dietary fiber; 4mg cholesterol; 591mg sodium; 359mg calcium; 18mg iron.

Lunch

Open-Faced Reuben Sandwich

2 slices reduced-calorie rye bread
$1^{1}/_2$ oz. lean corned beef, thinly sliced
$1/_2$ oz. reduced-fat Swiss cheese, sliced
black pepper, freshly ground

$1/_2$ tbsp. reduced-fat Thousand Island
   dressing
$1/_2$ cup sauerkraut, drained

Preheat broiler. Lightly toast bread. To assemble sandwiches, place toast slices onto rack in broiler pan; spread each slice with $1^{1}/_2$ tsp. dressing. Top each with $3/_4$ oz. corned beef, $1/_4$ cup sauerkraut, another $3/_4$ oz. corned beef and cheese. Sprinkle evenly with pepper to taste; broil 4 inches from heat for 2 minutes until cheese is melted and lightly browned. Serves 2.

Mustard Yogurt Dip: In a small bowl, combine $1/_4$ cup plain, nonfat yogurt and 2 tbsp. prepared mustard. Serve with $1/_2$ cup carrot sticks, $1/_2$ cup cauliflower florets and $1/_2$ cup sugar-free cherry-flavored gelatin mixed with fruit cocktail per person.

Nutritional Information: 456 calories (23% calories from fat); 12g fat; 24g protein; 67g carbohydrate; 12g dietary fiber; 30mg cholesterol; 1,827mg sodium; 397mg calcium; 6mg iron.

Dinner

Oriental Chicken and Cabbage Salad

1 cup canned, unsalted chicken broth
2 tsp. jalapeno chili, seeded and minced
4 large garlic cloves, minced
4 oz. snow peas, trimmed
$1/_4$ cup fresh cilantro, chopped
3 tbsp. minced fresh (or 1 tsp.
   ground) ginger

$1^{1}/_2$ lbs. skinless, boneless chicken
   breasts, cubed
$1/_3$ cup rice wine vinegar
1 tsp. sesame oil
1 (1-gram) packet sugar substitute
$4^{1}/_2$ cups red cabbage, sliced

2 cups mushrooms, sliced
2 tbsp. soy sauce, diluted with 2 tbsp. water
1^1/$_2$ cups carrots, grated

1 cup green onions, chopped
5^1/$_2$ cups Napa or green cabbage, sliced

Bring broth to simmer in heavy, large skillet over medium heat. Add chicken and simmer until cooked through, about 7 minutes. Transfer chicken to a bowl to cool. Add snow peas to broth and cook until tender, about 3 minutes. Using slotted spoon, transfer peas to bowl of cold water, then drain and set aside. Boil broth until reduced to ^{1}/$_3$ cup, about 7 minutes. Transfer to bowl; cool. Combine vinegar, chili, cilantro, soy sauce, ginger, garlic, sesame oil and sugar substitute in medium bowl. Add broth and whisk. Place cabbage, mushrooms, carrots and onions in large bowl. Add chicken. Top with dressing and toss to combine. (*Note:* May be made 6 hours ahead. Cover and refrigerate.) For a colorful presentation, serve salad in red cabbage leaves. Serve with ^{1}/$_4$ cup Chinese noodles per person. Serves 6.

Nutritional Information: 402 calories (25% calories from fat); 12g fat; 28g protein; 48g carbohydrate; 6g dietary fiber; 0mg cholesterol; 514mg sodium; 130mg calcium; 4mg iron.

HEALTHY SNACK OPTIONS

30 small pretzel sticks: 90 calories
6 *Lemon-Garlic Pita Chips*: 100 calories (see recipe below)
1 banana-chocolate whip (combine 1 cup fat-free milk, 1 small banana, a squeeze of chocolate syrup and a handful of ice cubes in a blender): 150 calories
3 cups air-popped popcorn sprinkled with 1 tablespoon parmesan cheese: 120 calories
1 *Peanut Butter Biscotti*: 125 calories (see recipe below)
1 mini-bagel with fat-free cream cheese (2 oz.): 145 calories
Snack Plate—25 red grapes, 3 tablespoons feta cheese, 6 crackers: 200 calories
Strawberry Malted Milk Shake: 250 calories (see recipe below)

SNACK RECIPES

Lemon-Garlic Pita Chips
3 (6-inch) pita bread rounds, split in half horizontally
2 teaspoons olive oil
1^1/$_2$ teaspoons lemon pepper
^{1}/$_4$ teaspoon garlic powder

Preheat oven to 400° F. Cut each pita half into 4 wedges; place on a baking sheet. Drizzle oil evenly over wedges. Combine lemon pepper and garlic powder; sprinkle evenly over wedges. Bake for 5 minutes or until crisp.

Nutritional Information: 146 calories (18% calories from fat); 3g fat; 4g protein; 26g carbohydrate; 1g dietary fiber; 0mg cholesterol; 369mg sodium: 39mg calcium; 1mg iron.

Peanut Butter Biscotti

2 cups all-purpose flour

$3/4$ teaspoon baking soda

$1/3$ cup chunky peanut butter

2 large eggs

Cooking spray

$3/4$ cup sugar

$1/4$ teaspoon salt

1 tsp. vanilla extract

2 large egg whites

Preheat oven to 325° F. Lightly spoon flour into dry measuring cups; level with a knife. Combine flour, sugar, baking soda and salt in a large bowl. Combine peanut butter, vanilla, eggs and egg whites in a medium bowl, stirring well with a whisk; add to flour mixture, stirring just until blended. Turn dough out onto a lightly floured surface; shape dough into a 10-inch-long roll. Place roll on a baking sheet coated with cooking spray and flatten to 1-inch thickness. Bake at 325° F for 35 minutes. Remove roll from baking sheet and cool 10 minutes on a wire rack. Reduce oven temperature to 300° F. Cut roll diagonally into 18 ($1/2$-inch) slices. Place slices, cut sides down, on baking sheet. Bake at 300° F for 20 minutes. Turn cookies over; bake an additional 20 minutes (cookies will be slightly soft in center but will harden as they cool). Remove from baking sheet; cool completely on a wire rack.

Nutritional Information: 125 calories (22% calories from fat); 3g fat; 4g protein; 20g carbohydrate; 1g dietary fiber; 24mg cholesterol; 119mg sodium; 7mg calcium; 1mg iron.

Strawberry Malted Milk Shake

2 cups vanilla low fat ice cream

$1^1/2$ cups halved strawberries

$1/4$ cup skim milk

3 tablespoons malted milk powder

1 tablespoon sugar

Whole strawberries with green caps (optional)

Place first 5 ingredients in a blender, and process until smooth. Garnish with whole strawberries, if desired. Serve immediately.

Nutritional Information: 250 calories (20% calories from fat); 6g fat; 7g protein; 45g carbohydrate; 2g dietary fiber; 16mg cholesterol; 175mg sodium; 213mg calcium: 1mg iron.

Member Survey

Please answer the following questions to help your leader plan your First Place 4 Health meetings so that your needs might be met in this session. Give this form to your leader at the first group meeting.

Name _____   Birth date _____

Please list those who live in your household.

Name	Relationship	Age

What church do you attend? _____

Are you interested in receiving more information about our church?

      Yes   No

Occupation _____

What talent or area of expertise would you be willing to share with our class?

_____

Why did you join First Place 4 Health?

_____

With notice, would you be willing to lead a Bible study discussion one week?

      Yes   No

Are you comfortable praying out loud? _____

If the assistant leader were absent, would you be willing to assist in weighing in members and possibly evaluating the Live It Trackers?

      Yes   No

Any other comments:

_____

_____

Personal Weight and Measurement Record

Week	Weight	+ or -	Goal this Session	Pounds to goal
1				
2				
3				
4				
5				
6				
7				
8				
9				
10				
11				
12				

Beginning Measurements

Waist _____ Hips _____ Thighs _____ Chest _____

Ending Measurements

Waist _____ Hips _____ Thighs _____ Chest _____

First Place 4 Health
Prayer Partner

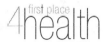

SEEK GOD
FIRST
Week
1

Date: _____

Name: _____

Home Phone: (_____) _____

Work Phone: (_____) _____

Email: _____

Personal Prayer Concerns:

_____

_____

_____

_____

_____

_____

This form is for prayer requests that are personal to you and your journey in First Place 4 Health. Please complete this form and have it ready to turn in when you arrive at your group meeting.

First Place 4 Health
Prayer Partner

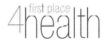

SEEK GOD
FIRST
Week
2

SCRIPTURE VERSE TO MEMORIZE FOR WEEK THREE:

If you believe, you will receive whatever you ask for in prayer.

MATTHEW 21:22

Date: _____

Name: _____

Home Phone: (_____) _____

Work Phone: (_____) _____

Email: _____

Personal Prayer Concerns:

_____

_____

_____

_____

_____

_____

This form is for prayer requests that are personal to you and your journey in First Place 4 Health. Please complete this form and have it ready to turn in when you arrive at your group meeting.

First Place 4 Health
Prayer Partner

4 first place
health

SEEK GOD
FIRST
Week
3

SCRIPTURE VERSE TO MEMORIZE FOR WEEK FOUR:

Whoever has my commands and obeys them, he is the one who loves me. He who loves me will be loved by my Father, and I too will love him and show myself to him.

JOHN 14:21

Date: _____

Name: _____

Home Phone: (_____) _____

Work Phone: (_____) _____

Email: _____

Personal Prayer Concerns:

_____

_____

_____

_____

_____

_____

_____

This form is for prayer requests that are personal to you and your journey in First Place 4 Health. Please complete this form and have it ready to turn in when you arrive at your group meeting.

First Place 4 Health
Prayer Partner

4 first place
health

SEEK GOD
FIRST
Week
4

SCRIPTURE VERSE TO MEMORIZE FOR WEEK FIVE:

You know my folly, O God; my guilt is not hidden from you.

PSALM 69:5

Date: _____

Name: _____

Home Phone: (___) _____

Work Phone: (___) _____

Email: _____

Personal Prayer Concerns:

_____

_____

_____

_____

_____

_____

_____

_____

This form is for prayer requests that are personal to you and your journey in First Place 4 Health. Please complete this form and have it ready to turn in when you arrive at your group meeting.

First Place 4 Health
Prayer Partner

4 first place
health

SEEK GOD
FIRST
Week
5

No temptation has seized you except what is common to man. And God is faithful;
he will not let you be tempted beyond what you can bear. But when you are tempted,
he will also provide a way out so that you can stand up under it.

1 CORINTHIANS 10:13

Date: _____

Name: _____

Home Phone: (_____)_____

Work Phone: (_____)_____

Email: _____

Personal Prayer Concerns:

_____

_____

_____

_____

_____

_____

_____

This form is for prayer requests that are personal to you and your journey in First Place 4 Health. Please complete this form and have it ready to turn in when you arrive at your group meeting.

First Place 4 Health
Prayer Partner

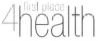

SEEK GOD
FIRST
Week
6

SCRIPTURE VERSE TO MEMORIZE FOR WEEK SEVEN:
Man does not live on bread alone,
but on every word that comes from the mouth of God.

MATTHEW 4:4

Date: _____

Name: _____

Home Phone: (_____) _____

Work Phone: (_____) _____

Email: _____

Personal Prayer Concerns:

_____

_____

_____

_____

_____

_____

This form is for prayer requests that are personal to you and your journey in First Place 4 Health. Please complete this form and have it ready to turn in when you arrive at your group meeting.

First Place 4 Health
Prayer Partner

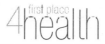

SEEK GOD
FIRST
Week
7

*Do not conform any longer to the pattern of this world, but be transformed by
the renewing of your mind. Then you will be able to test and approve what
God's will is—his good, pleasing and perfect will.*

ROMANS 12:2

Date: _____

Name: _____

Home Phone: (_____)

Work Phone: (_____)

Email: _____

Personal Prayer Concerns:

_____

_____

_____

_____

_____

_____

_____

This form is for prayer requests that are personal to you and your journey in First Place 4 Health. Please complete this
form and have it ready to turn in when you arrive at your group meeting.

First Place 4 Health
Prayer Partner

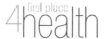

SEEK GOD
FIRST
Week
8

SCRIPTURE VERSE TO MEMORIZE FOR WEEK NINE:

Do you not know that your body is a temple of the Holy Spirit, who is in you, whom you have received from God? You are not your own; you were bought at a price. Therefore honor God with your body.

1 CORINTHIANS 6:19-20

Date: _____

Name: _____

Home Phone: ( ) _____

Work Phone: ( ) _____

Email: _____

Personal Prayer Concerns:

_____

_____

_____

_____

_____

_____

_____

This form is for prayer requests that are personal to you and your journey in First Place 4 Health. Please complete this form and have it ready to turn in when you arrive at your group meeting.

First Place 4 Health
Prayer Partner

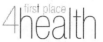

SEEK GOD
FIRST
Week
9

Date: _____

Name: _____

Home Phone: (_____)_____

Work Phone: (_____)_____

Email: _____

Personal Prayer Concerns:

_____

_____

_____

_____

_____

_____

_____

This form is for prayer requests that are personal to you and your journey in First Place 4 Health. Please complete this form and have it ready to turn in when you arrive at your group meeting.

First Place 4 Health
Prayer Partner

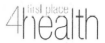

SEEK GOD
FIRST
Week
10

SCRIPTURE VERSE TO MEMORIZE FOR WEEK ELEVEN:

*A new command I give you: Love one another. As I have loved you,
so you must love one another. By this all men will know that you
are my disciples, if you love one another.*

JOHN 13:34-35

Date: _____

Name: _____

Home Phone: (_____)_____

Work Phone: (_____)_____

Email: _____

Personal Prayer Concerns:

_____

_____

_____

_____

_____

_____

_____

This form is for prayer requests that are personal to you and your journey in First Place 4 Health. Please complete this form and have it ready to turn in when you arrive at your group meeting.

First Place 4 Health
Prayer Partner

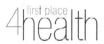

SEEK GOD
FIRST
Week
11

Date: _____

Name: _____

Home Phone: (_____) _____

Work Phone: (_____) _____

Email: _____

Personal Prayer Concerns:

_____

_____

_____

_____

_____

_____

_____

This form is for prayer requests that are personal to you and your journey in First Place 4 Health. Please complete this form and have it ready to turn in when you arrive at your group meeting.

Live It Tracker

Name: _____ Loss/gain: _____ lbs.

Date: _____ Week #: ____ Caloric Range: _____ My food goal for next week: _____

Activity Level: None, < 30 min/day, 30-60 min/day, 60+ min/day My activity goal for next week: _____

Group	Daily Calories							
	1300-1400	1500-1600	1700-1800	1900-2000	2100-2200	2300-2400	2500-2600	2700-2800
Fruits	1.5-2 c.	1.5-2 c.	1.5-2 c.	2-2.5 c.	2-2.5 c.	2.5-3.5 c.	3.5-4.5 c.	3.5-4.5 c.
Vegetables	1.5-2 c.	2-2.5 c.	2.5-3 c.	2.5-3 c.	3-3.5 c.	3.5-4.5 c.	4.5-5 c.	4.5-5 c.
Grains	5 oz-eq.	5-6 oz-eq.	6-7 oz-eq.	6-7 oz-eq.	7-8 oz-eq.	8-9 oz-eq.	9-10 oz-eq.	10-11 oz-eq.
Meat & Beans	4 oz-eq.	5 oz-eq.	5-5.5 oz-eq.	5.5-6.5 oz-eq.	6.5-7 oz-eq.	7-7.5 oz-eq.	7-7.5 oz-eq.	7.5-8 oz-eq.
Milk	2-3 c.	3 c.	3 c.	3 c.	3 c.	3 c.	3 c.	3 c.
Healthy Oils	4 tsp.	5 tsp.	5 tsp.	6 tsp.	6 tsp.	7 tsp.	8 tsp.	8 tsp.

Day/Date: _____

Breakfast: _____ Lunch: _____

Dinner: _____ Snack: _____

Group	Fruits	Vegetables	Grains	Meat & Beans	Milk	Oils
Goal Amount						
Estimate Your Total						
Increase ⇧ or Decrease? ⇩						

Physical Activity: _____ Spiritual Activity: _____

Steps/Miles/Minutes: _____

Day/Date: _____

Breakfast: _____ Lunch: _____

Dinner: _____ Snack: _____

Group	Fruits	Vegetables	Grains	Meat & Beans	Milk	Oils
Goal Amount						
Estimate Your Total						
Increase ⇧ or Decrease? ⇩						

Physical Activity: _____ Spiritual Activity: _____

Steps/Miles/Minutes: _____

Day/Date: _____

Breakfast: _____ Lunch: _____

Dinner: _____ Snack: _____

Group	Fruits	Vegetables	Grains	Meat & Beans	Milk	Oils
Goal Amount						
Estimate Your Total						
Increase ⇧ or Decrease? ⇩						

Physical Activity: _____ Spiritual Activity: _____

Steps/Miles/Minutes: _____

Day/Date: _____

Breakfast: _____ Lunch: _____

Dinner: _____ Snack: _____

Group	Fruits	Vegetables	Grains	Meat & Beans	Milk	Oils
Goal Amount						
Estimate Your Total						
Increase ⬆ or Decrease? ⬇						

Physical Activity: _____ Spiritual Activity: _____

Steps/Miles/Minutes: _____ _____

Day/Date: _____

Breakfast: _____ Lunch: _____

Dinner: _____ Snack: _____

Group	Fruits	Vegetables	Grains	Meat & Beans	Milk	Oils
Goal Amount						
Estimate Your Total						
Increase ⬆ or Decrease? ⬇						

Physical Activity: _____ Spiritual Activity: _____

Steps/Miles/Minutes: _____ _____

Day/Date: _____

Breakfast: _____ Lunch: _____

Dinner: _____ Snack: _____

Group	Fruits	Vegetables	Grains	Meat & Beans	Milk	Oils
Goal Amount						
Estimate Your Total						
Increase ⬆ or Decrease? ⬇						

Physical Activity: _____ Spiritual Activity: _____

Steps/Miles/Minutes: _____ _____

Day/Date: _____

Breakfast: _____ Lunch: _____

Dinner: _____ Snack: _____

Group	Fruits	Vegetables	Grains	Meat & Beans	Milk	Oils
Goal Amount						
Estimate Your Total						
Increase ⬆ or Decrease? ⬇						

Physical Activity: _____ Spiritual Activity: _____

Steps/Miles/Minutes: _____ _____

Live It Tracker

Name: _____ Loss/gain: _____ lbs.

Date: _____ Week #: _____ Calorie Range: _____ My food goal for next week: _____

Activity Level: None, < 30 min/day, 30-60 min/day, 60+ min/day My activity goal for next week: _____

Group	Daily Calories							
	1300-1400	1500-1600	1700-1800	1900-2000	2100-2200	2300-2400	2500-2600	2700-2800
Fruits	1.5-2 c.	1.5-2 c.	1.5-2 c.	2-2.5 c.	2-2.5 c.	2.5-3.5 c.	3.5-4.5 c.	3.5-4.5 c.
Vegetables	1.5-2 c.	2-2.5 c.	2.5-3 c.	2.5-3 c.	3-3.5 c.	3.5-4.5 c.	4.5-5 c.	4.5-5 c.
Grains	5 oz-eq.	5-6 oz-eq.	6-7 oz-eq.	6-7 oz-eq.	7-8 oz-eq.	8-9 oz-eq.	9-10 oz-eq.	10-11 oz-eq.
Meat & Beans	4 oz-eq.	5 oz-eq.	5-5.5 oz-eq.	5.5-6.5 oz-eq.	6.5-7 oz-eq.	7-7.5 oz-eq.	7-7.5 oz-eq.	7.5-8 oz-eq.
Milk	2-3 c.	3 c.	3 c.	3 c.	3 c.	3 c.	3 c.	3 c.
Healthy Oils	4 tsp.	5 tsp.	5 tsp.	6 tsp.	6 tsp.	7 tsp.	8 tsp.	8 tsp.

Day/Date:

Breakfast: _____ Lunch: _____

Dinner: _____ Snack: _____

Group	Fruits	Vegetables	Grains	Meat & Beans	Milk	Oils
Goal Amount						
Estimate Your Total						
Increase ⇧ or Decrease? ⇩						

Physical Activity: _____ Spiritual Activity: _____

Steps/Miles/Minutes: _____

Day/Date:

Breakfast: _____ Lunch: _____

Dinner: _____ Snack: _____

Group	Fruits	Vegetables	Grains	Meat & Beans	Milk	Oils
Goal Amount						
Estimate Your Total						
Increase ⇧ or Decrease? ⇩						

Physical Activity: _____ Spiritual Activity: _____

Steps/Miles/Minutes: _____

Day/Date:

Breakfast: _____ Lunch: _____

Dinner: _____ Snack: _____

Group	Fruits	Vegetables	Grains	Meat & Beans	Milk	Oils
Goal Amount						
Estimate Your Total						
Increase ⇧ or Decrease? ⇩						

Physical Activity: _____ Spiritual Activity: _____

Steps/Miles/Minutes: _____

Day/Date:

Breakfast: _____   Lunch: _____
_____
Dinner: _____   Snack: _____
_____

Group	Fruits	Vegetables	Grains	Meat & Beans	Milk	Oils
Goal Amount						
Estimate Your Total						
Increase ⬆ or Decrease? ⬇						

Physical Activity: _____   Spiritual Activity: _____
Steps/Miles/Minutes: _____   _____

Day/Date:

Breakfast: _____   Lunch: _____
_____
Dinner: _____   Snack: _____
_____

Group	Fruits	Vegetables	Grains	Meat & Beans	Milk	Oils
Goal Amount						
Estimate Your Total						
Increase ⬆ or Decrease? ⬇						

Physical Activity: _____   Spiritual Activity: _____
Steps/Miles/Minutes: _____   _____

Day/Date:

Breakfast: _____   Lunch: _____
_____
Dinner: _____   Snack: _____
_____

Group	Fruits	Vegetables	Grains	Meat & Beans	Milk	Oils
Goal Amount						
Estimate Your Total						
Increase ⬆ or Decrease? ⬇						

Physical Activity: _____   Spiritual Activity: _____
Steps/Miles/Minutes: _____   _____

Day/Date:

Breakfast: _____   Lunch: _____
_____
Dinner: _____   Snack: _____
_____

Group	Fruits	Vegetables	Grains	Meat & Beans	Milk	Oils
Goal Amount						
Estimate Your Total						
Increase ⬆ or Decrease? ⬇						

Physical Activity: _____   Spiritual Activity: _____
Steps/Miles/Minutes: _____   _____

Live It Tracker

Name: _____ Loss/gain: _____ lbs.

Date: _____ Week #: ____ Calorie Range: _____ My food goal for next week: _____

Activity Level: None, < 30 min/day, 30-60 min/day, 60+ min/day   My activity goal for next week: _____

Group	Daily Calories							
	1300-1400	1500-1600	1700-1800	1900-2000	2100-2200	2300-2400	2500-2600	2700-2800
Fruits	1.5-2 c.	1.5-2 c.	1.5-2 c.	2-2.5 c.	2-2.5 c.	2.5-3.5 c.	3.5-4.5 c.	3.5-4.5 c.
Vegetables	1.5-2 c.	2-2.5 c.	2.5-3 c.	2.5-3 c.	3-3.5 c.	3.5-4.5 c.	4.5-5 c.	4.5-5 c.
Grains	5 oz-eq.	5-6 oz-eq.	6-7 oz-eq.	6-7 oz-eq.	7-8 oz-eq.	8-9 oz-eq.	9-10 oz-eq.	10-11 oz-eq.
Meat & Beans	4 oz-eq.	5 oz-eq.	5-5.5 oz-eq.	5.5-6.5 oz-eq.	6.5-7 oz-eq.	7-7.5 oz-eq.	7-7.5 oz-eq.	7.5-8 oz-eq.
Milk	2-3 c.	3 c.	3 c.	3 c.	3 c.	3 c.	3 c.	3 c.
Healthy Oils	4 tsp.	5 tsp.	5 tsp.	6 tsp.	6 tsp.	7 tsp.	8 tsp.	8 tsp.

Day/Date: _____

Breakfast: _____ Lunch: _____

Dinner: _____ Snack: _____

Group	Fruits	Vegetables	Grains	Meat & Beans	Milk	Oils
Goal Amount						
Estimate Your Total						
Increase ⇧ or Decrease? ⇩						

Physical Activity: _____ Spiritual Activity: _____

Steps/Miles/Minutes: _____

Day/Date: _____

Breakfast: _____ Lunch: _____

Dinner: _____ Snack: _____

Group	Fruits	Vegetables	Grains	Meat & Beans	Milk	Oils
Goal Amount						
Estimate Your Total						
Increase ⇧ or Decrease? ⇩						

Physical Activity: _____ Spiritual Activity: _____

Steps/Miles/Minutes: _____

Day/Date: _____

Breakfast: _____ Lunch: _____

Dinner: _____ Snack: _____

Group	Fruits	Vegetables	Grains	Meat & Beans	Milk	Oils
Goal Amount						
Estimate Your Total						
Increase ⇧ or Decrease? ⇩						

Physical Activity: _____ Spiritual Activity: _____

Steps/Miles/Minutes: _____

Day/Date:

Breakfast: _____   Lunch: _____

Dinner: _____   Snack: _____

Group	Fruits	Vegetables	Grains	Meat & Beans	Milk	Oils
Goal Amount						
Estimate Your Total						
Increase ⇧ or Decrease? ⇩						

Physical Activity: _____   Spiritual Activity: _____

Steps/Miles/Minutes: _____   _____

Day/Date:

Breakfast: _____   Lunch: _____

Dinner: _____   Snack: _____

Group	Fruits	Vegetables	Grains	Meat & Beans	Milk	Oils
Goal Amount						
Estimate Your Total						
Increase ⇧ or Decrease? ⇩						

Physical Activity: _____   Spiritual Activity: _____

Steps/Miles/Minutes: _____   _____

Day/Date:

Breakfast: _____   Lunch: _____

Dinner: _____   Snack: _____

Group	Fruits	Vegetables	Grains	Meat & Beans	Milk	Oils
Goal Amount						
Estimate Your Total						
Increase ⇧ or Decrease? ⇩						

Physical Activity: _____   Spiritual Activity: _____

Steps/Miles/Minutes: _____   _____

Day/Date:

Breakfast: _____   Lunch: _____

Dinner: _____   Snack: _____

Group	Fruits	Vegetables	Grains	Meat & Beans	Milk	Oils
Goal Amount						
Estimate Your Total						
Increase ⇧ or Decrease? ⇩						

Physical Activity: _____   Spiritual Activity: _____

Steps/Miles/Minutes: _____   _____

Live It Tracker

Name: _____ Loss/gain: _____ lbs.

Date: _____ Week #: ____ Calorie Range: _____ My food goal for next week: _____

Activity Level: None, < 30 min/day, 30-60 min/day, 60+ min/day My activity goal for next week: _____

Group	Daily Calories							
	1300-1400	1500-1600	1700-1800	1900-2000	2100-2200	2300-2400	2500-2600	2700-2800
Fruits	1.5-2 c.	1.5-2 c.	1.5-2 c.	2-2.5 c.	2-2.5 c.	2.5-3.5 c.	3.5-4.5 c.	3.5-4.5 c.
Vegetables	1.5-2 c.	2-2.5 c.	2.5-3 c.	2.5-3 c.	3-3.5 c.	3.5-4.5 c.	4.5-5 c.	4.5-5 c.
Grains	5 oz-eq.	5-6 oz-eq.	6-7 oz-eq.	6-7 oz-eq.	7-8 oz-eq.	8-9 oz-eq.	9-10 oz-eq.	10-11 oz-eq.
Meat & Beans	4 oz-eq.	5 oz-eq.	5-5.5 oz-eq.	5.5-6.5 oz-eq.	6.5-7 oz-eq.	7-7.5 oz-eq.	7-7.5 oz-eq.	7.5-8 oz-eq.
Milk	2-3 c.	3 c.	3 c.	3 c.	3 c.	3 c.	3 c.	3 c.
Healthy Oils	4 tsp.	5 tsp.	5 tsp.	6 tsp.	6 tsp.	7 tsp.	8 tsp.	8 tsp.

Day/Date:

Breakfast: _____ Lunch: _____

Dinner: _____ Snack: _____

Group	Fruits	Vegetables	Grains	Meat & Beans	Milk	Oils
Goal Amount						
Estimate Your Total						
Increase ⇧ or Decrease? ⇩						

Physical Activity: _____ Spiritual Activity: _____

Steps/Miles/Minutes: _____

Day/Date:

Breakfast: _____ Lunch: _____

Dinner: _____ Snack: _____

Group	Fruits	Vegetables	Grains	Meat & Beans	Milk	Oils
Goal Amount						
Estimate Your Total						
Increase ⇧ or Decrease? ⇩						

Physical Activity: _____ Spiritual Activity: _____

Steps/Miles/Minutes: _____

Day/Date:

Breakfast: _____ Lunch: _____

Dinner: _____ Snack: _____

Group	Fruits	Vegetables	Grains	Meat & Beans	Milk	Oils
Goal Amount						
Estimate Your Total						
Increase ⇧ or Decrease? ⇩						

Physical Activity: _____ Spiritual Activity: _____

Steps/Miles/Minutes: _____

Day/Date:

Breakfast: _____ Lunch: _____

Dinner: _____ Snack: _____

Group	Fruits	Vegetables	Grains	Meat & Beans	Milk	Oils
Goal Amount						
Estimate Your Total						
Increase ⇧ or Decrease? ⇩						

Physical Activity: _____ Spiritual Activity: _____

Steps/Miles/Minutes: _____ _____

Day/Date:

Breakfast: _____ Lunch: _____

Dinner: _____ Snack: _____

Group	Fruits	Vegetables	Grains	Meat & Beans	Milk	Oils
Goal Amount						
Estimate Your Total						
Increase ⇧ or Decrease? ⇩						

Physical Activity: _____ Spiritual Activity: _____

Steps/Miles/Minutes: _____ _____

Day/Date:

Breakfast: _____ Lunch: _____

Dinner: _____ Snack: _____

Group	Fruits	Vegetables	Grains	Meat & Beans	Milk	Oils
Goal Amount						
Estimate Your Total						
Increase ⇧ or Decrease? ⇩						

Physical Activity: _____ Spiritual Activity: _____

Steps/Miles/Minutes: _____ _____

Day/Date:

Breakfast: _____ Lunch: _____

Dinner: _____ Snack: _____

Group	Fruits	Vegetables	Grains	Meat & Beans	Milk	Oils
Goal Amount						
Estimate Your Total						
Increase ⇧ or Decrease? ⇩						

Physical Activity: _____ Spiritual Activity: _____

Steps/Miles/Minutes: _____ _____

Live It Tracker

Name: _____ Loss/gain: _____ lbs.

Date: _____ Week #: _____ Calorie Range: _____ My food goal for next week: _____

Activity Level: None, < 30 min/day, 30-60 min/day, 60+ min/day   My activity goal for next week: _____

Group	Daily Calories							
	1300-1400	1500-1600	1700-1800	1900-2000	2100-2200	2300-2400	2500-2600	2700-2800
Fruits	1.5-2 c.	1.5-2 c.	1.5-2 c.	2-2.5 c.	2-2.5 c.	2.5-3.5 c.	3.5-4.5 c.	3.5-4.5 c.
Vegetables	1.5-2 c.	2-2.5 c.	2.5-3 c.	2.5-3 c.	3-3.5 c.	3.5-4.5 c.	4.5-5 c.	4.5-5 c.
Grains	5 oz-eq.	5-6 oz-eq.	6-7 oz-eq.	6-7 oz-eq.	7-8 oz-eq.	8-9 oz-eq.	9-10 oz-eq.	10-11 oz-eq.
Meat & Beans	4 oz-eq.	5 oz-eq.	5-5.5 oz-eq.	5.5-6.5 oz-eq.	6.5-7 oz-eq.	7-7.5 oz-eq.	7-7.5 oz-eq.	7.5-8 oz-eq.
Milk	2-3 c.	3 c.	3 c.	3 c.	3 c.	3 c.	3 c.	3 c.
Healthy Oils	4 tsp.	5 tsp.	5 tsp.	6 tsp.	6 tsp.	7 tsp.	8 tsp.	8 tsp.

Day/Date:

Breakfast: _____ Lunch: _____

Dinner: _____ Snack: _____

Group	Fruits	Vegetables	Grains	Meat & Beans	Milk	Oils
Goal Amount						
Estimate Your Total						
Increase ⇧ or Decrease? ⇩						

Physical Activity: _____ Spiritual Activity: _____

Steps/Miles/Minutes: _____

Day/Date:

Breakfast: _____ Lunch: _____

Dinner: _____ Snack: _____

Group	Fruits	Vegetables	Grains	Meat & Beans	Milk	Oils
Goal Amount						
Estimate Your Total						
Increase ⇧ or Decrease? ⇩						

Physical Activity: _____ Spiritual Activity: _____

Steps/Miles/Minutes: _____

Day/Date:

Breakfast: _____ Lunch: _____

Dinner: _____ Snack: _____

Group	Fruits	Vegetables	Grains	Meat & Beans	Milk	Oils
Goal Amount						
Estimate Your Total						
Increase ⇧ or Decrease? ⇩						

Physical Activity: _____ Spiritual Activity: _____

Steps/Miles/Minutes: _____

Day/Date: _____

Breakfast: _____ Lunch: _____

Dinner: _____ Snack: _____

Group	Fruits	Vegetables	Grains	Meat & Beans	Milk	Oils
Goal Amount						
Estimate Your Total						
Increase ⇧ or Decrease? ⇩						

Physical Activity: _____ Spiritual Activity: _____

Steps/Miles/Minutes: _____ _____

Day/Date: _____

Breakfast: _____ Lunch: _____

Dinner: _____ Snack: _____

Group	Fruits	Vegetables	Grains	Meat & Beans	Milk	Oils
Goal Amount						
Estimate Your Total						
Increase ⇧ or Decrease? ⇩						

Physical Activity: _____ Spiritual Activity: _____

Steps/Miles/Minutes: _____ _____

Day/Date: _____

Breakfast: _____ Lunch: _____

Dinner: _____ Snack: _____

Group	Fruits	Vegetables	Grains	Meat & Beans	Milk	Oils
Goal Amount						
Estimate Your Total						
Increase ⇧ or Decrease? ⇩						

Physical Activity: _____ Spiritual Activity: _____

Steps/Miles/Minutes: _____ _____

Day/Date: _____

Breakfast: _____ Lunch: _____

Dinner: _____ Snack: _____

Group	Fruits	Vegetables	Grains	Meat & Beans	Milk	Oils
Goal Amount						
Estimate Your Total						
Increase ⇧ or Decrease? ⇩						

Physical Activity: _____ Spiritual Activity: _____

Steps/Miles/Minutes: _____ _____

Live It Tracker

Name: _____ Loss/gain: _____ lbs.

Date: _____ Week #: ____ Calorie Range: _____ My food goal for next week: _____

Activity Level: None, < 30 min/day, 30-60 min/day, 60+ min/day My activity goal for next week: _____

Group	Daily Calories							
	1300-1400	1500-1600	1700-1800	1900-2000	2100-2200	2300-2400	2500-2600	2700-2800
Fruits	1.5-2 c.	1.5-2 c.	1.5-2 c.	2-2.5 c.	2-2.5 c.	2.5-3.5 c.	3.5-4.5 c.	3.5-4.5 c.
Vegetables	1.5-2 c.	2-2.5 c.	2.5-3 c.	2.5-3 c.	3-3.5 c.	3.5-4.5 c.	4.5-5 c.	4.5-5 c.
Grains	5 oz-eq.	5-6 oz-eq.	6-7 oz-eq.	6-7 oz-eq.	7-8 oz-eq.	8-9 oz-eq.	9-10 oz-eq.	10-11 oz-eq.
Meat & Beans	4 oz-eq.	5 oz-eq.	5-5.5 oz-eq.	5.5-6.5 oz-eq.	6.5-7 oz-eq.	7-7.5 oz-eq.	7-7.5 oz-eq.	7.5-8 oz-eq.
Milk	2-3 c.	3 c.	3 c.	3 c.	3 c.	3 c.	3 c.	3 c.
Healthy Oils	4 tsp.	5 tsp.	5 tsp.	6 tsp.	6 tsp.	7 tsp.	8 tsp.	8 tsp.

Day/Date:

Breakfast: _____ Lunch: _____

Dinner: _____ Snack: _____

Group	Fruits	Vegetables	Grains	Meat & Beans	Milk	Oils
Goal Amount						
Estimate Your Total						
Increase ⇧ or Decrease? ⇩						

Physical Activity: _____ Spiritual Activity: _____

Steps/Miles/Minutes: _____

Day/Date:

Breakfast: _____ Lunch: _____

Dinner: _____ Snack: _____

Group	Fruits	Vegetables	Grains	Meat & Beans	Milk	Oils
Goal Amount						
Estimate Your Total						
Increase ⇧ or Decrease? ⇩						

Physical Activity: _____ Spiritual Activity: _____

Steps/Miles/Minutes: _____

Day/Date:

Breakfast: _____ Lunch: _____

Dinner: _____ Snack: _____

Group	Fruits	Vegetables	Grains	Meat & Beans	Milk	Oils
Goal Amount						
Estimate Your Total						
Increase ⇧ or Decrease? ⇩						

Physical Activity: _____ Spiritual Activity: _____

Steps/Miles/Minutes: _____

Day/Date: _____

Breakfast: _____ Lunch: _____

Dinner: _____ Snack: _____

Group	Fruits	Vegetables	Grains	Meat & Beans	Milk	Oils
Goal Amount						
Estimate Your Total						
Increase ⬆ or Decrease? ⬇						

Physical Activity: _____ Spiritual Activity: _____

Steps/Miles/Minutes: _____

Day/Date: _____

Breakfast: _____ Lunch: _____

Dinner: _____ Snack: _____

Group	Fruits	Vegetables	Grains	Meat & Beans	Milk	Oils
Goal Amount						
Estimate Your Total						
Increase ⬆ or Decrease? ⬇						

Physical Activity: _____ Spiritual Activity: _____

Steps/Miles/Minutes: _____

Day/Date: _____

Breakfast: _____ Lunch: _____

Dinner: _____ Snack: _____

Group	Fruits	Vegetables	Grains	Meat & Beans	Milk	Oils
Goal Amount						
Estimate Your Total						
Increase ⬆ or Decrease? ⬇						

Physical Activity: _____ Spiritual Activity: _____

Steps/Miles/Minutes: _____

Day/Date: _____

Breakfast: _____ Lunch: _____

Dinner: _____ Snack: _____

Group	Fruits	Vegetables	Grains	Meat & Beans	Milk	Oils
Goal Amount						
Estimate Your Total						
Increase ⬆ or Decrease? ⬇						

Physical Activity: _____ Spiritual Activity: _____

Steps/Miles/Minutes: _____

Live It Tracker

Name: _____ Loss/gain: _____ lbs.

Date: _____ Week #: _____ Calorie Range: _____ My food goal for next week: _____

Activity Level: None, < 30 min/day, 30-60 min/day, 60+ min/day My activity goal for next week: _____

Group	Daily Calories							
	1300-1400	1500-1600	1700-1800	1900-2000	2100-2200	2300-2400	2500-2600	2700-2800
Fruits	1.5-2 c.	1.5-2 c.	1.5-2 c.	2-2.5 c.	2-2.5 c.	2.5-3.5 c.	3.5-4.5 c.	3.5-4.5 c.
Vegetables	1.5-2 c.	2-2.5 c.	2.5-3 c.	2.5-3 c.	3-3.5 c.	3.5-4.5 c.	4.5-5 c.	4.5-5 c.
Grains	5 oz-eq.	5-6 oz-eq.	6-7 oz-eq.	6-7 oz-eq.	7-8 oz-eq.	8-9 oz-eq.	9-10 oz-eq.	10-11 oz-eq.
Meat & Beans	4 oz-eq.	5 oz-eq.	5-5.5 oz-eq.	5.5-6.5 oz-eq.	6.5-7 oz-eq.	7-7.5 oz-eq.	7-7.5 oz-eq.	7.5-8 oz-eq.
Milk	2-3 c.	3 c.	3 c.	3 c.	3 c.	3 c.	3 c.	3 c.
Healthy Oils	4 tsp.	5 tsp.	5 tsp.	6 tsp.	6 tsp.	7 tsp.	8 tsp.	8 tsp.

Day/Date: _____

Breakfast: _____ Lunch: _____

Dinner: _____ Snack: _____

Group	Fruits	Vegetables	Grains	Meat & Beans	Milk	Oils
Goal Amount						
Estimate Your Total						
Increase ⇧ or Decrease? ⇩						

Physical Activity: _____ Spiritual Activity: _____

Steps/Miles/Minutes: _____

Day/Date: _____

Breakfast: _____ Lunch: _____

Dinner: _____ Snack: _____

Group	Fruits	Vegetables	Grains	Meat & Beans	Milk	Oils
Goal Amount						
Estimate Your Total						
Increase ⇧ or Decrease? ⇩						

Physical Activity: _____ Spiritual Activity: _____

Steps/Miles/Minutes: _____

Day/Date: _____

Breakfast: _____ Lunch: _____

Dinner: _____ Snack: _____

Group	Fruits	Vegetables	Grains	Meat & Beans	Milk	Oils
Goal Amount						
Estimate Your Total						
Increase ⇧ or Decrease? ⇩						

Physical Activity: _____ Spiritual Activity: _____

Steps/Miles/Minutes: _____

Day/Date:

Breakfast: _____ Lunch: _____

Dinner: _____ Snack: _____

Group	Fruits	Vegetables	Grains	Meat & Beans	Milk	Oils
Goal Amount						
Estimate Your Total						
Increase ⬆ or Decrease? ⬇						

Physical Activity: _____ Spiritual Activity: _____

Steps/Miles/Minutes: _____ _____

Day/Date:

Breakfast: _____ Lunch: _____

Dinner: _____ Snack: _____

Group	Fruits	Vegetables	Grains	Meat & Beans	Milk	Oils
Goal Amount						
Estimate Your Total						
Increase ⬆ or Decrease? ⬇						

Physical Activity: _____ Spiritual Activity: _____

Steps/Miles/Minutes: _____ _____

Day/Date:

Breakfast: _____ Lunch: _____

Dinner: _____ Snack: _____

Group	Fruits	Vegetables	Grains	Meat & Beans	Milk	Oils
Goal Amount						
Estimate Your Total						
Increase ⬆ or Decrease? ⬇						

Physical Activity: _____ Spiritual Activity: _____

Steps/Miles/Minutes: _____ _____

Day/Date:

Breakfast: _____ Lunch: _____

Dinner: _____ Snack: _____

Group	Fruits	Vegetables	Grains	Meat & Beans	Milk	Oils
Goal Amount						
Estimate Your Total						
Increase ⬆ or Decrease? ⬇						

Physical Activity: _____ Spiritual Activity: _____

Steps/Miles/Minutes: _____ _____

Live It Tracker

Name: _____ Loss/gain: _____ lbs.

Date: _____ Week #: ____ Caloric Range: _____ My food goal for next week: _____

Activity Level: None, < 30 min/day, 30-60 min/day, 60+ min/day My activity goal for next week: _____

Group	Daily Calories							
	1300-1400	1500-1600	1700-1800	1900-2000	2100-2200	2300-2400	2500-2600	2700-2800
Fruits	1.5-2 c.	1.5-2 c.	1.5-2 c.	2-2.5 c.	2-2.5 c.	2.5-3.5 c.	3.5-4.5 c.	3.5-4.5 c.
Vegetables	1.5-2 c.	2-2.5 c.	2.5-3 c.	2.5-3 c.	3-3.5 c.	3.5-4.5 c.	4.5-5 c.	4.5-5 c.
Grains	5 oz-eq.	5-6 oz-eq.	6-7 oz-eq.	6-7 oz-eq.	7-8 oz-eq.	8-9 oz-eq.	9-10 oz-eq.	10-11 oz-eq.
Meat & Beans	4 oz-eq.	5 oz-eq.	5-5.5 oz-eq.	5.5-6.5 oz-eq.	6.5-7 oz-eq.	7-7.5 oz-eq.	7-7.5 oz-eq.	7.5-8 oz-eq.
Milk	2-3 c.	3 c.	3 c.	3 c.	3 c.	3 c.	3 c.	3 c.
Healthy Oils	4 tsp.	5 tsp.	5 tsp.	6 tsp.	6 tsp.	7 tsp.	8 tsp.	8 tsp.

Day/Date:

Breakfast: _____ Lunch: _____

Dinner: _____ Snack: _____

Group	Fruits	Vegetables	Grains	Meat & Beans	Milk	Oils
Goal Amount						
Estimate Your Total						
Increase ⇧ or Decrease? ⇩						

Physical Activity: _____ Spiritual Activity: _____

Steps/Miles/Minutes: _____ _____

Day/Date:

Breakfast: _____ Lunch: _____

Dinner: _____ Snack: _____

Group	Fruits	Vegetables	Grains	Meat & Beans	Milk	Oils
Goal Amount						
Estimate Your Total						
Increase ⇧ or Decrease? ⇩						

Physical Activity: _____ Spiritual Activity: _____

Steps/Miles/Minutes: _____ _____

Day/Date:

Breakfast: _____ Lunch: _____

Dinner: _____ Snack: _____

Group	Fruits	Vegetables	Grains	Meat & Beans	Milk	Oils
Goal Amount						
Estimate Your Total						
Increase ⇧ or Decrease? ⇩						

Physical Activity: _____ Spiritual Activity: _____

Steps/Miles/Minutes: _____ _____

Breakfast: _____ Lunch: _____

Dinner: _____ Snack: _____

Group	Fruits	Vegetables	Grains	Meat & Beans	Milk	Oils
Goal Amount						
Estimate Your Total						
Increase ⬆ or Decrease? ⬇						

Physical Activity: _____ Spiritual Activity: _____

Steps/Miles/Minutes: _____ _____

Breakfast: _____ Lunch: _____

Dinner: _____ Snack: _____

Group	Fruits	Vegetables	Grains	Meat & Beans	Milk	Oils
Goal Amount						
Estimate Your Total						
Increase ⬆ or Decrease? ⬇						

Physical Activity: _____ Spiritual Activity: _____

Steps/Miles/Minutes: _____ _____

Breakfast: _____ Lunch: _____

Dinner: _____ Snack: _____

Group	Fruits	Vegetables	Grains	Meat & Beans	Milk	Oils
Goal Amount						
Estimate Your Total						
Increase ⬆ or Decrease? ⬇						

Physical Activity: _____ Spiritual Activity: _____

Steps/Miles/Minutes: _____ _____

Breakfast: _____ Lunch: _____

Dinner: _____ Snack: _____

Group	Fruits	Vegetables	Grains	Meat & Beans	Milk	Oils
Goal Amount						
Estimate Your Total						
Increase ⬆ or Decrease? ⬇						

Physical Activity: _____ Spiritual Activity: _____

Steps/Miles/Minutes: _____ _____

Live It Tracker

Name: _____ Loss/gain: _____ lbs.

Date: _____ Week #: _____ Calorie Range: _____ My food goal for next week: _____

Activity Level: None, < 30 min/day, 30-60 min/day, 60+ min/day My activity goal for next week: _____

Group	Daily Calories							
	1300-1400	1500-1600	1700-1800	1900-2000	2100-2200	2300-2400	2500-2600	2700-2800
Fruits	1.5-2 c.	1.5-2 c.	1.5-2 c.	2-2.5 c.	2-2.5 c.	2.5-3.5 c.	3.5-4.5 c.	3.5-4.5 c.
Vegetables	1.5-2 c.	2-2.5 c.	2.5-3 c.	2.5-3 c.	3-3.5 c.	3.5-4.5 c.	4.5-5 c.	4.5-5 c.
Grains	5 oz-eq.	5-6 oz-eq.	6-7 oz-eq.	6-7 oz-eq.	7-8 oz-eq.	8-9 oz-eq.	9-10 oz-eq.	10-11 oz-eq.
Meat & Beans	4 oz-eq.	5 oz-eq.	5-5.5 oz-eq.	5.5-6.5 oz-eq.	6.5-7 oz-eq.	7-7.5 oz-eq.	7-7.5 oz-eq.	7.5-8 oz-eq.
Milk	2-3 c.	3 c.	3 c.	3 c.	3 c.	3 c.	3 c.	3 c.
Healthy Oils	4 tsp.	5 tsp.	5 tsp.	6 tsp.	6 tsp.	7 tsp.	8 tsp.	8 tsp.

Day/Date:

Breakfast: _____ Lunch: _____

Dinner: _____ Snack: _____

Group	Fruits	Vegetables	Grains	Meat & Beans	Milk	Oils
Goal Amount						
Estimate Your Total						
Increase ⇧ or Decrease? ⇩						

Physical Activity: _____ Spiritual Activity: _____

Steps/Miles/Minutes: _____

Day/Date:

Breakfast: _____ Lunch: _____

Dinner: _____ Snack: _____

Group	Fruits	Vegetables	Grains	Meat & Beans	Milk	Oils
Goal Amount						
Estimate Your Total						
Increase ⇧ or Decrease? ⇩						

Physical Activity: _____ Spiritual Activity: _____

Steps/Miles/Minutes: _____

Day/Date:

Breakfast: _____ Lunch: _____

Dinner: _____ Snack: _____

Group	Fruits	Vegetables	Grains	Meat & Beans	Milk	Oils
Goal Amount						
Estimate Your Total						
Increase ⇧ or Decrease? ⇩						

Physical Activity: _____ Spiritual Activity: _____

Steps/Miles/Minutes: _____

Day/Date:

Breakfast: _____   Lunch: _____

Dinner: _____   Snack: _____

Group	Fruits	Vegetables	Grains	Meat & Beans	Milk	Oils
Goal Amount						
Estimate Your Total						
Increase ⇧ or Decrease? ⇩						

Physical Activity: _____   Spiritual Activity: _____

Steps/Miles/Minutes: _____   _____

Day/Date:

Breakfast: _____   Lunch: _____

Dinner: _____   Snack: _____

Group	Fruits	Vegetables	Grains	Meat & Beans	Milk	Oils
Goal Amount						
Estimate Your Total						
Increase ⇧ or Decrease? ⇩						

Physical Activity: _____   Spiritual Activity: _____

Steps/Miles/Minutes: _____   _____

Day/Date:

Breakfast: _____   Lunch: _____

Dinner: _____   Snack: _____

Group	Fruits	Vegetables	Grains	Meat & Beans	Milk	Oils
Goal Amount						
Estimate Your Total						
Increase ⇧ or Decrease? ⇩						

Physical Activity: _____   Spiritual Activity: _____

Steps/Miles/Minutes: _____   _____

Day/Date:

Breakfast: _____   Lunch: _____

Dinner: _____   Snack: _____

Group	Fruits	Vegetables	Grains	Meat & Beans	Milk	Oils
Goal Amount						
Estimate Your Total						
Increase ⇧ or Decrease? ⇩						

Physical Activity: _____   Spiritual Activity: _____

Steps/Miles/Minutes: _____   _____

Live It Tracker

Name: _____ Loss/gain: _____ lbs.

Date: _____ Week #: ____ Caloric Range: _____ My food goal for next week: _____

Activity Level: None, < 30 min/day, 30-60 min/day, 60+ min/day My activity goal for next week: _____

Group	Daily Calories							
	1300-1400	1500-1600	1700-1800	1900-2000	2100-2200	2300-2400	2500-2600	2700-2800
Fruits	1.5-2 c.	1.5-2 c.	1.5-2 c.	2-2.5 c.	2-2.5 c.	2.5-3.5 c.	3.5-4.5 c.	3.5-4.5 c.
Vegetables	1.5-2 c.	2-2.5 c.	2.5-3 c.	2.5-3 c.	3-3.5 c.	3.5-4.5 c.	4.5-5 c.	4.5-5 c.
Grains	5 oz-eq.	5-6 oz-eq.	6-7 oz-eq.	6-7 oz-eq.	7-8 oz-eq.	8-9 oz-eq.	9-10 oz-eq.	10-11 oz-eq.
Meat & Beans	4 oz-eq.	5 oz-eq.	5-5.5 oz-eq.	5.5-6.5 oz-eq.	6.5-7 oz-eq.	7-7.5 oz-eq.	7-7.5 oz-eq.	7.5-8 oz-eq.
Milk	2-3 c.	3 c.	3 c.	3 c.	3 c.	3 c.	3 c.	3 c.
Healthy Oils	4 tsp.	5 tsp.	5 tsp.	6 tsp.	6 tsp.	7 tsp.	8 tsp.	8 tsp.

Day/Date:

Breakfast: _____   Lunch: _____

Dinner: _____   Snack: _____

Group	Fruits	Vegetables	Grains	Meat & Beans	Milk	Oils
Goal Amount						
Estimate Your Total						
Increase ⬆ or Decrease? ⬇						

Physical Activity: _____   Spiritual Activity: _____

Steps/Miles/Minutes: _____   _____

Day/Date:

Breakfast: _____   Lunch: _____

Dinner: _____   Snack: _____

Group	Fruits	Vegetables	Grains	Meat & Beans	Milk	Oils
Goal Amount						
Estimate Your Total						
Increase ⬆ or Decrease? ⬇						

Physical Activity: _____   Spiritual Activity: _____

Steps/Miles/Minutes: _____   _____

Day/Date:

Breakfast: _____   Lunch: _____

Dinner: _____   Snack: _____

Group	Fruits	Vegetables	Grains	Meat & Beans	Milk	Oils
Goal Amount						
Estimate Your Total						
Increase ⬆ or Decrease? ⬇						

Physical Activity: _____   Spiritual Activity: _____

Steps/Miles/Minutes: _____   _____

Day/Date:

Breakfast: _____ Lunch: _____

Dinner: _____ Snack: _____

Group	Fruits	Vegetables	Grains	Meat & Beans	Milk	Oils
Goal Amount						
Estimate Your Total						
Increase ⬆ or Decrease? ⬇						

Physical Activity: _____ Spiritual Activity: _____

Steps/Miles/Minutes: _____ _____

Day/Date:

Breakfast: _____ Lunch: _____

Dinner: _____ Snack: _____

Group	Fruits	Vegetables	Grains	Meat & Beans	Milk	Oils
Goal Amount						
Estimate Your Total						
Increase ⬆ or Decrease? ⬇						

Physical Activity: _____ Spiritual Activity: _____

Steps/Miles/Minutes: _____ _____

Day/Date:

Breakfast: _____ Lunch: _____

Dinner: _____ Snack: _____

Group	Fruits	Vegetables	Grains	Meat & Beans	Milk	Oils
Goal Amount						
Estimate Your Total						
Increase ⬆ or Decrease? ⬇						

Physical Activity: _____ Spiritual Activity: _____

Steps/Miles/Minutes: _____ _____

Day/Date:

Breakfast: _____ Lunch: _____

Dinner: _____ Snack: _____

Group	Fruits	Vegetables	Grains	Meat & Beans	Milk	Oils
Goal Amount						
Estimate Your Total						
Increase ⬆ or Decrease? ⬇						

Physical Activity: _____ Spiritual Activity: _____

Steps/Miles/Minutes: _____ _____

Live It Tracker

Name: _____ Loss/gain: _____ lbs.

Date: _____ Week #: _____ Calorie Range: _____ My food goal for next week: _____

Activity Level: None, < 30 min/day, 30-60 min/day, 60+ min/day My activity goal for next week: _____

Group	Daily Calories							
	1300-1400	1500-1600	1700-1800	1900-2000	2100-2200	2300-2400	2500-2600	2700-2800
Fruits	1.5-2 c.	1.5-2 c.	1.5-2 c.	2-2.5 c.	2-2.5 c.	2.5-3.5 c.	3.5-4.5 c.	3.5-4.5 c.
Vegetables	1.5-2 c.	2-2.5 c.	2.5-3 c.	2.5-3 c.	3-3.5 c.	3.5-4.5 c.	4.5-5 c.	4.5-5 c.
Grains	5 oz-eq.	5-6 oz-eq.	6-7 oz-eq.	6-7 oz-eq.	7-8 oz-eq.	8-9 oz-eq.	9-10 oz-eq.	10-11 oz-eq.
Meat & Beans	4 oz-eq.	5 oz-eq.	5-5.5 oz-eq.	5.5-6.5 oz-eq.	6.5-7 oz-eq.	7-7.5 oz-eq.	7-7.5 oz-eq.	7.5-8 oz-eq.
Milk	2-3 c.	3 c.	3 c.	3 c.	3 c.	3 c.	3 c.	3 c.
Healthy Oils	4 tsp.	5 tsp.	5 tsp.	6 tsp.	6 tsp.	7 tsp.	8 tsp.	8 tsp.

Day/Date:

Breakfast: _____ Lunch: _____

Dinner: _____ Snack: _____

Group	Fruits	Vegetables	Grains	Meat & Beans	Milk	Oils
Goal Amount						
Estimate Your Total						
Increase ⇧ or Decrease? ⇩						

Physical Activity: _____ Spiritual Activity: _____

Steps/Miles/Minutes: _____

Day/Date:

Breakfast: _____ Lunch: _____

Dinner: _____ Snack: _____

Group	Fruits	Vegetables	Grains	Meat & Beans	Milk	Oils
Goal Amount						
Estimate Your Total						
Increase ⇧ or Decrease? ⇩						

Physical Activity: _____ Spiritual Activity: _____

Steps/Miles/Minutes: _____

Day/Date:

Breakfast: _____ Lunch: _____

Dinner: _____ Snack: _____

Group	Fruits	Vegetables	Grains	Meat & Beans	Milk	Oils
Goal Amount						
Estimate Your Total						
Increase ⇧ or Decrease? ⇩						

Physical Activity: _____ Spiritual Activity: _____

Steps/Miles/Minutes: _____

Day/Date: _____

Breakfast: _____ Lunch: _____

Dinner: _____ Snack: _____

Group	Fruits	Vegetables	Grains	Meat & Beans	Milk	Oils
Goal Amount						
Estimate Your Total						
Increase ⇧ or Decrease? ⇩						

Physical Activity: _____ Spiritual Activity: _____

Steps/Miles/Minutes: _____ _____

Day/Date: _____

Breakfast: _____ Lunch: _____

Dinner: _____ Snack: _____

Group	Fruits	Vegetables	Grains	Meat & Beans	Milk	Oils
Goal Amount						
Estimate Your Total						
Increase ⇧ or Decrease? ⇩						

Physical Activity: _____ Spiritual Activity: _____

Steps/Miles/Minutes: _____ _____

Day/Date: _____

Breakfast: _____ Lunch: _____

Dinner: _____ Snack: _____

Group	Fruits	Vegetables	Grains	Meat & Beans	Milk	Oils
Goal Amount						
Estimate Your Total						
Increase ⇧ or Decrease? ⇩						

Physical Activity: _____ Spiritual Activity: _____

Steps/Miles/Minutes: _____ _____

Day/Date: _____

Breakfast: _____ Lunch: _____

Dinner: _____ Snack: _____

Group	Fruits	Vegetables	Grains	Meat & Beans	Milk	Oils
Goal Amount						
Estimate Your Total						
Increase ⇧ or Decrease? ⇩						

Physical Activity: _____ Spiritual Activity: _____

Steps/Miles/Minutes: _____ _____

Live It Tracker

Name: _____ Loss/gain: _____ lbs.

Date: _____ Week #: ____ Calorie Range: _____ My food goal for next week: _____

Activity Level: None, < 30 min/day, 30-60 min/day, 60+ min/day My activity goal for next week: _____

Group	Daily Calories							
	1300-1400	1500-1600	1700-1800	1900-2000	2100-2200	2300-2400	2500-2600	2700-2800
Fruits	1.5-2 c.	1.5-2 c.	1.5-2 c.	2-2.5 c.	2-2.5 c.	2.5-3.5 c.	3.5-4.5 c.	3.5-4.5 c.
Vegetables	1.5-2 c.	2-2.5 c.	2.5-3 c.	2.5-3 c.	3-3.5 c.	3.5-4.5 c.	4.5-5 c.	4.5-5 c.
Grains	5 oz-eq.	5-6 oz-eq.	6-7 oz-eq.	6-7 oz-eq.	7-8 oz-eq.	8-9 oz-eq.	9-10 oz-eq.	10-11 oz-eq.
Meat & Beans	4 oz-eq.	5 oz-eq.	5-5.5 oz-eq.	5.5-6.5 oz-eq.	6.5-7 oz-eq.	7-7.5 oz-eq.	7-7.5 oz-eq.	7.5-8 oz-eq.
Milk	2-3 c.	3 c.	3 c.	3 c.	3 c.	3 c.	3 c.	3 c.
Healthy Oils	4 tsp.	5 tsp.	5 tsp.	6 tsp.	6 tsp.	7 tsp.	8 tsp.	8 tsp.

Day/Date:

Breakfast: _____   Lunch: _____

Dinner: _____   Snack: _____

Group	Fruits	Vegetables	Grains	Meat & Beans	Milk	Oils
Goal Amount						
Estimate Your Total						
Increase ⇧ or Decrease? ⇩						

Physical Activity: _____   Spiritual Activity: _____

Steps/Miles/Minutes: _____

Day/Date:

Breakfast: _____   Lunch: _____

Dinner: _____   Snack: _____

Group	Fruits	Vegetables	Grains	Meat & Beans	Milk	Oils
Goal Amount						
Estimate Your Total						
Increase ⇧ or Decrease? ⇩						

Physical Activity: _____   Spiritual Activity: _____

Steps/Miles/Minutes: _____

Day/Date:

Breakfast: _____   Lunch: _____

Dinner: _____   Snack: _____

Group	Fruits	Vegetables	Grains	Meat & Beans	Milk	Oils
Goal Amount						
Estimate Your Total						
Increase ⇧ or Decrease? ⇩						

Physical Activity: _____   Spiritual Activity: _____

Steps/Miles/Minutes: _____

Day/Date:

Breakfast: _____ Lunch: _____

Dinner: _____ Snack: _____

Group	Fruits	Vegetables	Grains	Meat & Beans	Milk	Oils
Goal Amount						
Estimate Your Total						
Increase ⇧ or Decrease? ⇩						

Physical Activity: _____ Spiritual Activity: _____

Steps/Miles/Minutes: _____

Day/Date:

Breakfast: _____ Lunch: _____

Dinner: _____ Snack: _____

Group	Fruits	Vegetables	Grains	Meat & Beans	Milk	Oils
Goal Amount						
Estimate Your Total						
Increase ⇧ or Decrease? ⇩						

Physical Activity: _____ Spiritual Activity: _____

Steps/Miles/Minutes: _____

Day/Date:

Breakfast: _____ Lunch: _____

Dinner: _____ Snack: _____

Group	Fruits	Vegetables	Grains	Meat & Beans	Milk	Oils
Goal Amount						
Estimate Your Total						
Increase ⇧ or Decrease? ⇩						

Physical Activity: _____ Spiritual Activity: _____

Steps/Miles/Minutes: _____

Day/Date:

Breakfast: _____ Lunch: _____

Dinner: _____ Snack: _____

Group	Fruits	Vegetables	Grains	Meat & Beans	Milk	Oils
Goal Amount						
Estimate Your Total						
Increase ⇧ or Decrease? ⇩						

Physical Activity: _____ Spiritual Activity: _____

Steps/Miles/Minutes: _____

let's count our miles!

Join the 100-Mile Club this Session

Can't walk that mile yet? Don't be discouraged! There are exercises you can do
to strengthen your body and burn those extra calories. Keep a record on your
Live It Tracker of the number of minutes you do these common physical activities, convert those minutes to miles following the chart below, and then mark
off each mile you have completed on the chart found on the back of the front
cover. Report your miles to your 100-Mile Club representative when you first
arrive each week. Remember, you are not competing with anyone else . . . just
yourself. Your job is to strive to reach 100 miles before the last meeting in this
session. You can do it—just keep on moving!

Walking
slowly, 2 mph	30 min. = 156 cal. = 1 mile
moderately, 3 mph	20 min. = 156 cal. = 1 mile
very briskly, 4 mph	15 min. = 156 cal. = 1 mile
speed walking	10 min. = 156 cal. = 1 mile
up stairs	13 min. = 159 cal. = 1 mile

Running/Jogging
10 min. = 156 cal. = 1 mile

Cycling Outdoors
slowly, <10 mph	20 min. = 156 cal. = 1 mile
light effort, 10-12 mph	12 min. = 156 cal. = 1 mile
moderate effort, 12-14 mph	10 min. = 156 cal. = 1 mile
vigorous effort, 14-16 mph	7.5 min. = 156 cal. = 1 mile
very fast, 16-19 mph	6.5 min. = 152 cal. = 1 mile

Sports Activities
Playing tennis (singles)	10 min. = 156 cal. = 1 mile
Swimming	
light to moderate effort	11 min. = 152 cal. = 1 mile
fast, vigorous effort	7.5 min. = 156 cal. = 1 mile
Softball	15 min. = 156 cal. = 1 mile
Golf	20 min. = 156 cal = 1 mile
Rollerblading	6.5 min. = 152 cal. = 1 mile
Ice skating	11 min. = 152 cal. = 1 mile

Jumping rope   7.5 min. = 156 cal. = 1 mile
Basketball   12 min. = 156 cal. = 1 mile
Soccer (casual)   15 min. = 159 cal. = 1 mile

Around the House
Mowing grass   22 min. = 156 cal. = 1 mile
Mopping, sweeping, vacuuming   19.5 min. = 155 cal. = 1 mile
Cooking   40 min. =160 cal. = 1 mile
Gardening   19 min. = 156 cal. = 1 mile
Housework (general)   35 min. = 156 cal. = 1 mile
Ironing   45 min. = 153 cal. = 1 mile
Raking leaves   25 min. = 150 cal. = 1 mile
Washing car   23 min. = 156 cal. = 1 mile
Washing dishes   45 min. = 153 cal. = 1 mile

At the Gym
Stair machine   8.5 min. = 155 cal. = 1 mile
Stationary bike
  slowly, 10 mph   30 min. = 156 cal. = 1 mile
  moderately, 10-13 mph   15 min. = 156 cal. = 1 mile
  vigorously, 13-16 mph   7.5 min. = 156 cal. = 1 mile
  briskly, 16-19 mph   6.5 min. = 156 cal. = 1 mile
Elliptical trainer   12 min. = 156 cal. = 1 mile
Weight machines (used vigorously)   13 min. = 152 cal.=1 mile
Aerobics
  low impact   15 min. = 156 cal. = 1 mile
  high impact   12 min. = 156 cal. = 1 mile
  water   20 min. = 156 cal. = 1 mile
Pilates   15 min. = 156 cal. = 1 mile
Raquetball (casual)   15 min. = 159 cal. = 1 mile
Stretching exercises   25 min. = 150 cal. = 1 mile
Weight lifting (also works for weight
  machines used moderately or gently)   30 min. = 156 cal. = 1 mile

Family Leisure
Playing piano   37 min. = 155 cal. = 1 mile
Jumping rope   10 min. = 152 cal. = 1 mile
Skating (moderate)   20 min. = 152 cal. = 1 mile
Swimming
  moderate   17 min. = 156 cal. = 1 mile
  vigorous   10 min. = 148 cal. = 1 mile
Table tennis   25 min. = 150 cal. = 1 mile
Walk/run/play with kids   25 min. = 150 cal. = 1 mile